W9-BWX-890

What You Need to Know about the Flu

Recent Titles in
Inside Diseases and Disorders

What You Need to Know about Autism
Christopher M. Cumo

What You Need to Know about ADHD
Victor B. Stolberg

What You Need to Know about ALS
Harry LeVine III

What You Need to Know about Eating Disorders
Jessica Bartley and Melissa Streno

What You Need to Know about Diabetes
Tish Davidson

What You Need to Know about the Flu

R. K. Devlin

Inside Diseases and Disorders

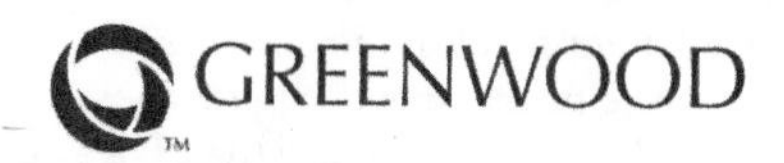

An Imprint of ABC-CLIO, LLC
Santa Barbara, California • Denver, Colorado

Library of Congress Cataloging-in-Publication Data

Names: Devlin, Roni K., 1968- author.
Title: What you need to know about the flu / R. K. Devlin.
Description: Santa Barbara, California : Greenwood, [2021] | Series: Inside diseases and disorders | Includes bibliographical references and index.
Identifiers: LCCN 2020018708 (print) | LCCN 2020018709 (ebook) | ISBN 9781440870071 (hardcover) | ISBN 9781440870088 (ebook)
Subjects: LCSH: Influenza.
Classification: LCC RC150 .D47 2021 (print) | LCC RC150 (ebook) | DDC 616.2/03—dc23
LC record available at https://lccn.loc.gov/2020018708
LC ebook record available at https://lccn.loc.gov/2020018709

ISBN: 978-1-4408-7007-1 (print)
978-1-4408-7008-8 (ebook)

25 24 23 22 21 1 2 3 4 5

This book is also available as an eBook.

Greenwood
An Imprint of ABC-CLIO, LLC

ABC-CLIO, LLC
147 Castilian Drive
Santa Barbara, California 93117
www.abc-clio.com

This book is printed on acid-free paper ∞

Manufactured in the United States of America

This book discusses treatments (including types of medication and other therapies), diagnostic tests for various symptoms and other disorders, and organizations. The author has made every effort to present accurate and up-to-date information. However, the information in this book is not intended to recommend or endorse particular treatments or organizations, or substitute for the care or medical advice of a qualified health professional, or to be used to alter any medical therapy without a medical doctor's advice. Specific situations may require specific therapeutic approaches not included in this book. For those reasons, we recommend that readers follow the advice of qualified health care professionals directly involved in their care. Readers who suspect they may have specific medical problems should consult a physician about any suggestions made in this book.

Contents

Series Foreword

Disease is as old as humanity itself, and it has been the leading cause of death and disability throughout history. From the Black Death in the Middle Ages to smallpox outbreaks among Native Americans to the modern-day epidemics of diabetes and heart disease, humans have lived with—and died from—all manner of ailments, whether caused by infectious agents, environmental and lifestyle factors, or genetic abnormalities. The field of medicine has been driven forward by our desire to combat and prevent disease and to improve the lives of those living with debilitating disorders. And while we have made great strides forward, particularly in the last 100 years, it is doubtful that mankind will ever be completely free of the burden of disease.

Greenwood's Inside Diseases and Disorders series examines some of the key diseases and disorders, both physical and psychological, affecting the world today. Some (such as diabetes, cardiovascular disease, and ADHD) have been selected because of their prominence within modern America. Others (such as Ebola, celiac disease, and autism) have been chosen because they are often discussed in the media and, in some cases, are controversial or the subject of scientific or cultural debate.

Because this series covers so many different diseases and disorders, we have striven to create uniformity across all books. To maximize clarity and consistency, each book in the series follows the same format. Each begins with a collection of frequently asked questions about the disease or disorder, followed by clear, concise answers. Chapter 1 provides a general introduction to the disease or disorder, including statistical information such as prevalence rates and demographic trends. The history of the disease or disorder, including how our understanding of it has evolved over time, is addressed in chapter 2. Chapter 3 examines causes and risk factors, whether genetic, microbial, or environmental, while chapter 4 discusses signs and symptoms. Chapter 5 covers the issues of diagnosis (and misdiagnosis), treatment, and management (whether with drugs, medical procedures, or lifestyle changes). How such treatment, or the lack thereof, affects a patient's long-term prognosis, as well as the risk of complications, are the subject of chapter 6. Chapter 7 explores the disease or disorder's effects on the friends and family of a patient—a dimension often overlooked in discussions of physical and psychological ailments. Chapter 8 discusses prevention strategies, while chapter 9 explores key issues or controversies, whether medical or sociocultural. Finally, chapter 10 profiles cutting-edge research and speculates on how things might change in the next few decades.

Each volume also features five fictional case studies to illustrate different aspects of the book's subject matter, highlighting key concepts and themes that have been explored throughout the text. The reader will also find a glossary of terms and a collection of print and electronic resources for additional information and further study.

As a final caveat, please be aware that the information presented in these books is no substitute for consultation with a licensed health care professional. These books do not claim to provide medical advice or guidance.

Introduction

Hippocrates (460–375 BCE) was a Greek physician and teacher who is now known as the "Father of Medicine." In 412 BCE, in the *Book of Epidemics,* Hippocrates was thought to be one of the first to describe an illness suggestive of influenza. He noted a flu-like syndrome called "fever of Perinthus" or "cough of Perinthus," which described a winter and a spring epidemic of an upper respiratory tract infection that occurred regularly every year at a port town called Perinthus, located in the northern part of Greece that is now Turkey. Other similar descriptions of a sickness thought to be influenza have been found written on paper dating back to the Middle Ages. In the fifteenth century, the term *influenza* originated in Italy for the first time to describe this episodic, but recurrent, clinical syndrome attributed to the "influence of the stars"; the word was adopted into English in the eighteenth century. Today, people across the globe often refer to it simply as the flu. The disease, by whatever name, and the germ that causes it, is the topic of this book.

Despite all we now know about the influenza virus and the infectious disease it causes, it remains a source of tremendous grief for humankind. Every year, influenza circulates through small towns and cities alike all across the globe as a seasonal infection. It's estimated that influenza infects between 5 and 15 percent of the world's population each year, with even higher numbers in children (about 30 percent). These statistics suggest that *every person* will be infected or exposed to the flu virus by the time they are four years old. A more recent study looking at seasonal flu between 2010 and 2018 in the United States has shown that the virus resulted in up to 23 million medical visits, almost a million hospitalizations, and up to 79,000 respiratory and circulatory deaths *each year.* Worldwide, it has been estimated that up to 645,000 respiratory deaths are associated with influenza annually.

While these statistics of severe disease and death are shockingly impressive, there are other consequences of influenza that are often overlooked: lost productivity from missed days at work, sky-high costs of medical care, and other economic burdens. One study that looked at the consequences of influenza in the United States based on the 2003 population found that direct medical costs averaged $10.4 billion annually, projected lost earnings due to illness and death amounted to $16.3 billion each year, and the total economic burden of annual influenza epidemics reached $87.1 billion.

Much has been discovered about the influenza virus since it was identified as a pathogen in the 1930s. Yet, even with all that is known about influenza and its potential for catastrophic consequences, there remains the struggle to prevent influenza and break the cycle of seasonal outbreaks, epidemics, and even pandemics. The virus is virulent, contagious, and prone to mutation; these characteristics make it difficult to control. According to the Centers for Disease Control and Prevention (CDC), the 2017–2018 influenza season was the first to be classified as "high severity" across all age groups. In addition to the high levels of outpatient clinic and emergency room visits, high rates of influenza-related hospitalizations, and impressive spread geographically, it was also one of the longest influenza seasons in recent years (although updated analysis now suggests the 2018–2019 flu season might have been even longer). In the United States, almost a million people were hospitalized during the 2017–2018 flu season, and nearly 80,000 people died. The number of cases of influenza-associated illness that occurred during the season (almost 50 million people) was the highest since the influenza pandemic of 2009.

With greater numbers of ill patients during the annual flu season, medical resources are stretched to the limit. The CDC noted that the number of hospitalizations during the 2017–2018 flu season exceeded the number of staffed hospital beds in the United States. Yet, it is considered fairly certain that a significant worldwide pandemic of influenza will occur sometime in the future, and it is clear that our health care systems may not be prepared for this sort of challenge—a pandemic could come with a global death toll that might be almost unimaginable.

It is not surprising, then, that measures to prevent, control, and treat influenza are being aggressively pursued. Considerable research is ongoing with regard to both prevention and treatment of the flu with medications and vaccinations. It is the goal of this book to help the reader understand influenza as a pathogen, a disease process, and both a personal and societal burden. It is only with full understanding that we can properly protect ourselves and our loved ones from the potential consequences of influenza well into the future.

Essential Questions

1. WHAT SORT OF GERM CAUSES THE FLU?

The germ that causes the flu is not a bacterium, nor a fungus or parasite. Rather, it is a virus. Viruses differ from the other types of germs because they are not considered by most scientists to be alive: they do not eat, drink, have sex, or produce waste. They are simply genetic material surrounded by a protective shell. In the case of the influenza virus, its unique outer envelope and enclosed genetic material allow it to infect the cells of the respiratory system and gain entry into the cells in order to make more viral particles, which are then released through respiratory secretions to infect other humans.

2. IS THERE A DIFFERENCE BETWEEN SEASONAL FLU AND "BIRD FLU"?

Seasonal flu occurs year after year in humans and is often due to influenza strains that have been around for a long time. For example, H1N1 is the virus that caused an influenza pandemic in 1918 and then circulated for 39 years; now, a new variation on that virus, pH1N1, has been in circulation for the last 10 years. The H3N2 viruses have been with us for 51 years and still cocirculate with the pH1N1 strains every season. "Bird flu," on the other hand, refers to infection caused by an entirely new strain of influenza due to antigenic shift, a process in which animal influenza viruses (such as those found in birds) and human influenza viruses initiate a "combined infection" in a cell of a species in which they can both multiply. These novel viral strains theoretically allow infectivity in humans, but with the presence of animal glycoproteins to which the majority of the human population has never before been exposed (and thus has no antibodies or immune protection). It is this sort of virus that has caused influenza pandemics in the past (and is expected to cause a flu pandemic in the future, too).

3. HOW DO PEOPLE CATCH THE FLU?

First, people who are infected with influenza can release small virus-containing droplets into the air when they cough, sneeze, or talk. These droplets can land in the mouths or noses or be breathed in by people who are around them (even up to six feet away!), and then the virus can infect the respiratory tract of its new host. Another way that influenza is spread from person to person is through contaminated respiratory secretions on hands and other surfaces; these secretions can be spread by hands to other people, especially if the hands come in contact with the mouth, nose, or eyes.

4. WHAT SYMPTOMS WILL I FEEL IF I BECOME INFECTED WITH THE FLU VIRUS?

In uncomplicated influenza infection, the most prominent symptoms are both systemic (triggered by the immune response) and localized (within the upper respiratory tract), including fever, shaking chills, headache, muscle aches, fatigue, congestion of the nose, sore throat, and cough. Though rare in occurrence, some people infected with influenza can experience symptoms involving an organ system beyond the lungs, such as inflammation of the heart, altered thinking, eye infection, kidney or liver injury, or toxic shock syndrome. Those infected with the flu can also develop secondary bacterial pneumonia.

5. IF I THINK I MIGHT HAVE THE FLU, SHOULD I GO TO MY DOCTOR?

Many people can (and should) manage their influenza illness at home; this practice helps prevent spread of the flu to others and allows rest needed for recovery. There are some symptoms that would prompt medical attention, however, including difficulty breathing, not being able to eat or drink (which can lead to dehydration), relapse of symptoms after an initial period of resolution (which might indicate a secondary infection with bacteria), or severe mental alterations. If influenza is highly suspected or proven by laboratory testing and if certain criteria are met, it is possible that your medical provider might be give you a prescription for antiviral medications to treat the flu.

6. HOW SICK CAN PATIENTS WITH THE FLU REALLY GET?

Most people who become infected with the flu have an uncomplicated course and recover without any serious consequences after a few days of illness. Infrequently, people infected with influenza will have symptoms in organ systems beyond the lungs. For some unfortunate people, however, infection with the flu virus can lead to primary viral pneumonia or development of secondary bacterial pneumonia; these lung complications are much more worrisome in terms of severity, often prompting a need for medical attention and raising the risk of death. Some humans are especially at risk for severe flu infections, including children under 5 years of age, people with chronic diseases, adults 65 years of age or older, immunocompromised people, pregnant women, and American Indians and Alaska Natives.

7. IF I'M SICK WITH THE FLU, WILL I PASS IT ON TO MY FRIENDS AND FAMILY?

When you are infected with the influenza virus, droplets of respiratory secretions, laden with viral particles, are sent into the air when you sneeze, cough, or even talk. They don't remain suspended in the air for long and travel less than three feet in most circumstances. Since these droplets can then enter the respiratory tract of a new host (either directly or by hands that have come in contact with surfaces contaminated with droplets), you can certainly pass the flu on to your friends and family. There are ways you can try to minimize your chance of spreading the flu to others: (a) cover your nose and mouth with a tissue when you cough or sneeze and then throw your tissues in the trash after you use it; (b) if you don't have a tissue available, cough or sneeze into your upper arm; (c) wash your hands often with soap and water or use an alcohol-based hand rub; d) try to limit your contact with other people while you're ill.

8. IS THERE ANYTHING I CAN DO TO AVOID GETTING THE FLU?

There are basic personal hygiene techniques and everyday preventative actions that can limit your chance of exposure to the flu virus, such as learning to not touch your face, keeping up with vigilant hand washing, cleaning and disinfecting surfaces and objects that may be contaminated with germs, and avoiding close contact with sick people. In some specific circumstances, use of antiviral medications for chemoprophylaxis may be indicated to prevent influenza infection. However, the best way to avoid getting the flu is to get the influenza vaccine *every year.* Vaccination not only offers a chance at prevention of the flu, but studies have shown that it also halves the risk for influenza-related hospitalization in adults and reduces the risk for pediatric deaths from influenza by 65 percent among healthy children and by 51 percent among children with high-risk medical conditions.

9. CAN I CATCH THE FLU FROM THE FLU VACCINE?

This is a common misperception, but no, you can't catch the flu from the flu vaccine. There are several different types of influenza vaccines (killed virus, cell culture based, recombinant, and live virus). In each of these vaccines, the viral strains are either inactivated (rendered "dead"), synthetically raised so that they are unable to replicate, or attenuated to be "cold adapted" in order to inhibit replication in the human body. Some people who have a vigorous immune reaction to the vaccine may experience flu-like symptoms, but these are not due to infection; rather, they are the manifestations of immune system activation.

10. IS THERE ANYTHING THAT CAN STOP A MAJOR FLU PANDEMIC FROM HAPPENING IN THE FUTURE?

Unfortunately, most scientists believe that another flu pandemic is inevitable. Despite the medical advances we've made in the last century, the likelihood of pandemics has actually increased because of greater human and avian/swine populations, global travel and integration, changes in land use, more exploitation of the natural environment, and the anti-vaccination movement. While coronaviruses are a different class of viruses than influenza, the 2020 COVID-19 pandemic illustrates just how quickly a new strain of a disease can spread and how devastating the consequences can be. The next influenza pandemic will be difficult to predict, so preparedness is the key to mitigation of the pandemic and recovery beyond its global course.

1

What Is Influenza?

Humankind has always struggled to perfectly understand the cause of mental and physical symptoms of illness. Early physicians and healers blamed ill humors, dirty air, or even the gods for the sicknesses that plagued their patients; treatments that attempted to maintain harmony of the humors, cleanse the dirty air, or placate the gods were, not surprisingly, of limited success. Fortunately, over time, dedicated and meticulous scientific research (and sometimes, surprising and unexpected discoveries) led to the identification of germs, including the specific virus that causes the flu. With greater understanding of the influenza virus, research could then focus on ways to both prevent and treat it.

DEFINITION OF A VIRUS

A researcher named Charles Chamberland (1851–1908), a colleague of Louis Pasteur (1822–1895), changed everything about our understanding of germs with the invention of a relatively simple, unglazed porcelain filter. This filter was able to trap bacteria but allowed smaller infectious particles to pass through. Botanists first using the filter found that diseases could be transmitted to plants by inoculating healthy specimens with the liquid that remained after filtration of samples from infected plants; the small particles in this filtrate were initially called *Contagium vivum fluidum,* meaning "soluble living germ." Ultimately, these germs became known as viruses, based on Latin for "venom" or "poisonous emanation." With further study, researchers were eventually able to show that viruses were not only the cause of diseases in plants but also responsible for many human illnesses like polio and yellow fever. It was only a matter of time, of course, until a virus was also discovered as the cause of influenza.

Unless you've studied microbiology, you might not be entirely sure what type of germs are responsible for certain infectious diseases. Bacteria are living one-celled organisms that make their own food, are often motile, and are able to reproduce. Examples of bacteria include *Staphylococcus aureus* and *Escherichia coli*. Fungi are organisms that were formally classified as plants, but they lack chlorophyll; fungi include molds, rusts, mildews, smuts, mushrooms, and yeasts. Parasites live in, with, or on another organism; examples of parasites that cause trouble for humans are the *Plasmodium* species, which cause malaria, and *Pediculus humanus capitis*, otherwise known as head lice. Viruses, on the other hand, are not considered by most scientists to be alive. They do not eat, drink, have sex, or produce waste. They are simply genetic material surrounded by a protective shell. Examples of human diseases caused by viruses include chicken pox, polio, AIDS, and, of course, influenza.

The exact origin of viruses on earth is not known. There are several theories that might explain their existence, though. One hypothesis suggests that viruses may be the result of "escaped" pieces of genetic material that originally came from a living organism. A second idea is that viruses were derived from living cells that "devolved," or reverted back to a more primitive form, through a process known as reverse evolution. Another view suggests that viruses originated as a primitive molecule capable of replication, or production of more molecules, implying that more advanced life forms could have evolved from them. Regardless of its origin, a viral particle (often called a virion) essentially exists for one purpose: to make more viruses. Despite this being its primary goal, viruses do not have sex; this means they are not able to reproduce on their own. They must invade the cells of a host and use the replicating machinery within the cells to make new viral particles. A virus, then, is a carrier for genes, nicely surrounded by a protective layer that can come in a variety of shapes; it is this shape that allows for identification of four main categories of viruses: helical, icosahedral, enveloped, and complex. Influenza is an enveloped virus.

Interestingly, in addition to allowing the virion to reach the desired cell type that it prefers to infect, the surrounding coat actually plays a role in determining how a virus might be transmitted between hosts, too. Coats that are made of fats are easily broken down outside of the body, so viruses with this type of shell must be transmitted with the aid of respiratory secretions, blood, or body fluid. For example, influenza can be spread from person to person in droplets that are expelled during coughing, sneezing, or even talking. Viruses without this type of outer packaging are more stable outside of their host and are usually transmitted by a route that is known as fecal-oral. This route requires that a host come in contact with fecal matter (on unwashed hands or food, for instance) and then transmit the virus, hiding in the fecal material, to their mouth. From there, the virus gets ingested and then travels to its desired location in the body to start its disease process. Examples of diseases caused by viruses that are transmitted via the fecal-oral route are polio and certain types of hepatitis.

The genetic material that is protected by the outer coat of the viral particle can come in a variety of shapes and sizes; it is made of either ribonucleic acid (RNA) or deoxyribonucleic acid (DNA). RNA and DNA are both strands of genes that encode for proteins, but there are subtle differences in the types of chemicals that make up their backbones. RNA and DNA are composed of units called nucleotides, which consist of a nitrogen base, a sugar, and a phosphate. RNA utilizes ribose sugars and four possible bases: adenine, guanine, cytosine, and uracil. DNA, conversely, uses deoxyribose sugars and adenine, guanine, cytosine, and thymine as its bases. While both RNA and DNA carry genetic instructions, DNA must be copied into a complementary RNA before proteins can be produced; this process is known as transcription. Once transcription has occurred, then translation, or production of proteins from the genetic code found in the RNA copy, can proceed. It is the specific sequence of the nucleotides within the RNA and DNA that acts as a blueprint for the production of proteins that are unique to a virus. The smallest viruses contain genes that will encode only a few different proteins, while larger viruses might have the ability to encode several hundred proteins. With its genetic material and the resulting proteins, a virus uses its host cell's replication pathways to make more viral particles, which then can infect other host cells and thereby cause ill effects. The purpose of this replication cycle, of course, is to allow ongoing production and survival of its kind, which is a reasonable goal for any infectious agent. With regard to ongoing existence, then, influenza may be considered a very successful virus. Indeed, it has caused seasonal outbreaks for centuries.

THE INFLUENZA VIRAL PARTICLE

Given that influenza has an amazing ability to persist as a pathogen, there must be certain characteristics of the viral particle that allow it to cause recurrent disease in animals and humans year after year. Medical technology has now advanced enough for researchers to classify the influenza virus in terms of its size, shape, and function.

Classification

Influenza belongs to a larger family of viruses called *Orthomyxoviridae*, and there are four types of influenza viruses, named in order of their discovery: A, B, C, and D. There are some similarities between each of the influenza viruses. However, they all have distinct characteristics, including how the genetic material is organized within the virion, the overall viral structure, the preference of the virus for a certain type of host, the seasonal characteristics, and the constellation of symptoms exhibited by those who become infected. Besides humans, many animals may catch or transmit the influenza virus, including pigs (swine), birds, seals, whales, and horses. However, it is the bird (avian) population that is most concerning when discussing the potential dangers of influenza for humans. In birds, influenza A causes a gastrointestinal infection that often is of little consequence to its avian host; this allows the virus to replicate and be excreted in high concentrations. The avian reservoir is large, active, and mobile, and the influenza virus is along for the ride wherever the bird populations may travel.

Characteristics

The diameter of an influenza virus is approximately 80–120 nanometers, so it can best be seen with the aid of an electron microscope. It can exist either in the form of a sphere or as elongated filamentous particles. Each influenza A and B viral particle has genetic material in the form of single-stranded RNA in eight separate segments; this RNA encodes for eight different proteins, each of which has a specific function. Six of these proteins are dedicated to viral reproduction, while the remaining two are responsible for the outer coat, which consists of spikes formed of glycoproteins (a class of proteins that have carbohydrate groups attached). With influenza A, the spikes contain either hemagglutinin (HA) or neuraminidase (NA), along with the protein M2. Influenza A is divided into subtypes based on these glycoproteins; there are 18 different HA subtypes and 11 different NA subtypes. See Figure 1.1 for a depiction of an influenza A viral particle. In contrast, influenza B has fixed HA and NA and thus is not divided into subtypes; however, there are two distinct lineages of the influenza B virus that circulate among the human population. Also, unlike influenza A (which has three proteins in its envelope), the influenza B virions have four proteins in the outer envelope. Influenza C is different from either influenza A or B, as it has only seven genome segments and its surface carries only one glycoprotein called hemagglutinin-esterase-fusion (HEF), which essentially functions as both HA and NA. These viral particles have hexagonal structures on the surface and form long, cordlike

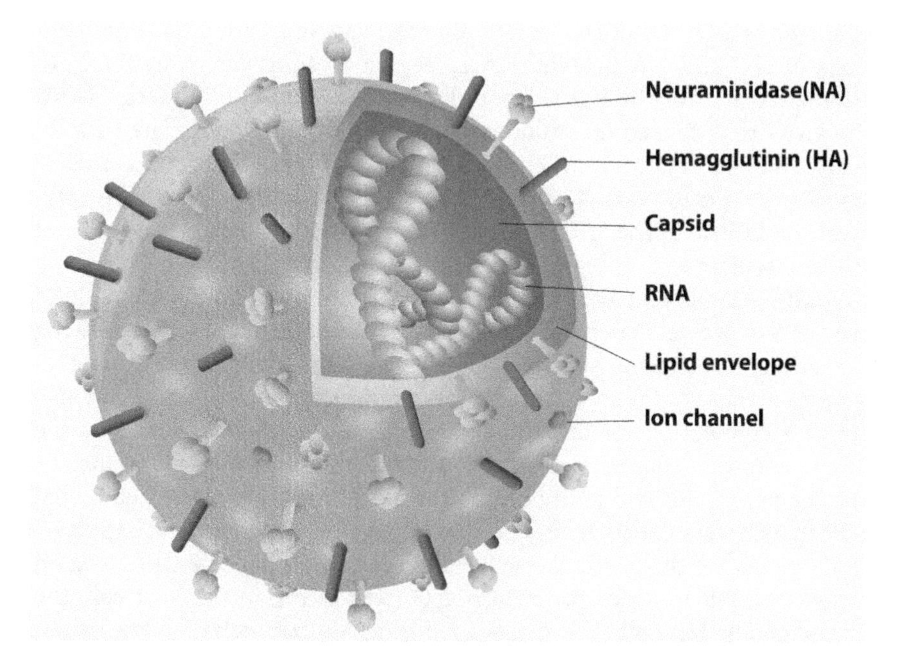

Figure 1.1 Structure of the Influenza A Virion (© Designua/Dreamstime.com)

shapes as they leave a host cell. Influenza D has the same genome structure as influenza C (seven RNA gene segments), and it also carries an HEF glycoprotein on its surface.

It is now known that influenza C can infect both humans and swine, and reassorted (mutated) viruses have been detected. However, despite the fact that nearly all adults have likely been infected with influenza C, it is not the cause of significant consequences in humans. Usually, infection with influenza C results in a mild upper respiratory illness; lower respiratory tract complications, such as pneumonia, are rare. Influenza D primarily infects cattle and has not been known to result in disease in humans. By far, influenza A is the most troublesome strain and will be the primary topic of discussion in this book.

The HA and NA glycoproteins have allowed scientists to define strains of influenza A in different species of mammals; the HA and NA also determine how infectious a flu strain might be for humans. Given that the type of HA and NA ultimately influences how dangerous a flu virus might be to humankind, identification of the HA and NA glycoproteins is necessary when attempting to predict, prevent, control, and treat influenza. The full name of an influenza virus requires the type (usually A or B), the host species (usually left out if the host is human), geographical site, serial number, year of isolation, and, finally, the HA and NA variants in parentheses. So, a fully identified avian influenza strain might be *A/goose/*

Guangdong/1/96 (H5N1). Despite all of the various potential combinations of HA and NA proteins, there are fewer subtypes consistently in circulation within the human population than you would guess. H1N1, the virus that caused an influenza pandemic in 1918, circulated for 39 years, and now, a new variation on that virus, pH1N1, has been in circulation for the last 10 years. Viruses belonging to the H2N2 strain were prevalent for 11 years. The H3N2 viruses have been with us for 51 years and still cocirculate with the pH1N1 strains every season.

Both HA and NA have very specific functions. The main portion of the HA protein projects outward from the viral envelope like a spike, allowing five different antigenic sites to be presented; this means that the spikes have an attraction for specific receptors on the cells of a host and can also act as a connection for antibodies, which are proteins produced by the immune system that help neutralize infectious agents. More specifically, HA binds to sialic acid found on the surface of respiratory tract epithelial cells in a process called adsorption and then enters the cell. If it can't perfectly penetrate the particular cell it targets, the flu particle will move on to another cell in order to try again. Once it is inside the host cell, the virion (and its HA spike) undergoes a shift in position, which allows shedding of the viral envelope. With the envelope no longer protecting it, the viral genetic material spills into the cell, and the RNA strands move into the host cell's nucleus. Then, the genetic material of the influenza RNA is processed via the host cell's machinery to produce proteins. These proteins are then packaged into new viral particles. Amazingly, it only takes about 6–10 hours for viral replication to occur.

The NA glycoprotein appears to be necessary for full penetration of the virion through the host's mucus layer, which lines the respiratory tract. Perhaps more importantly, though, NA enables a newly created viral particle to separate from the host cell. NA accomplishes this function specifically by cleaving sialic acid receptors from the HA molecule, from other NA proteins, and from glycoproteins and glycolipids at the host cell surface. If NA didn't allow this separation to occur, new viral particles produced during replication wouldn't be able to travel onward along the respiratory tract to infect new cells or to leave the host completely to infect others.

Virulence Factors

To be successful, a pathogen needs to be transmitted from host to host to perpetuate its existence, but without completely destroying its host population for good (which could ultimately render it nonexistent). Influenza seems pretty perfect in this respect: it can infect millions of hosts and has managed to survive for centuries. How, then, does the influenza virus manage to be so effective, and what factors contribute to its virulence? Clearly, the HA and NA glycoproteins are both key to the influenza virus's success. They allow recognition of the viral particle by the target host cell, attachment to the host cell's surface, penetration into the cell to allow viral replication, and assistance when new viral particles need to leave the cell. Thankfully, some of the current strains of avian influenza are not likely to cause human disease because they don't have perfect separation of HA when new viral particles try to move beyond their host cell. Another factor that helps in the success of the flu virus is sequestration: the proteins encoded by the influenza virus help hide the viral RNA. If the viral RNA isn't recognized by the host cell, then the host's immune system response might stall, and the virus can continue to replicate unchecked. In addition, during the late phase of infection, the influenza virus is able to monopolize the machinery of its host cell by shifting the focus of protein production to only those glycoproteins needed to make more viral particles (in contrast, an uninfected cell might produce hundreds of different glycoproteins).

During its replication process, the influenza virus kills its host cell by a number of different mechanisms: it decreases the host cell's ability to make its own proteins, degrades the host cell's genetic material so that it doesn't transcribe normally, and allows further breakdown of cellular proteins. While the cell is dying, the newly replicated influenza virions are more easily released. This process does take time, and usually, 18–72 hours have passed between the entry of the virus into the host cell and the onset of identifiable symptoms caused by cell death and the initiation of the immune and inflammatory response; this is known as the incubation period. Another mechanism that allows effective spread of the influenza virus from host to host is viral shedding. During the incubation period, the virus can be detected in the respiratory secretions of infected people before they show any obvious symptoms or realize that they are ill. The number of viral particles produced during an infection increases to a peak fairly rapidly beyond the incubation period and remains elevated for 24–48 hours and then decreases to low levels. Usually, an infected person can shed the influenza virus for 5–10 days (although certain special populations of people can shed virus for longer periods of time). The severity of a patient's symptoms seems to correlate with the amount of viral shedding as well.

While all of these virulence factors are impressive, perhaps the most frightening aspect of influenza's success as a pathogen lies in its ability to undergo mutation and to move from an animal source (like birds) to a human host. It is this tendency for mutation that prevents lifelong immunity to influenza with either infection or vaccination and leads to the increasing concern about a future pandemic from viral strains that originated in animals. Further details about mutation of the influenza virus will be discussed in chapter 3.

EPIDEMIOLOGY OF INFLUENZA

Epidemiology refers to the incidence, distribution, and control of a disease in a population, and with regard to influenza, it is truly fascinating. Influenza has a remarkable history as a virus through time, and it has shaped the history of humankind on a global scale. When considering the epidemiology of influenza, it is important to understand the terminology used to describe the disease manifestations with regard to human populations.

Outbreaks and Epidemics

An outbreak refers to the occurrence of a large number of cases of influenza in a short period of time. Outbreaks of influenza are common and occur yearly in many places across the globe. An epidemic refers to an outbreak that is confined to one location, such as a city or a country. Both influenza A and influenza B viruses cause seasonal epidemics. While many people recover easily from infection during seasonal flu outbreaks and epidemics, the virus still causes an impressive number of complications and deaths every year. As mentioned in the introduction to this book, one study looking at seasonal flu between 2010 and 2018 in the United States noted that the virus resulted in up to 23 million medical visits, almost a million hospitalizations, and up to 79,000 respiratory and circulatory deaths *each year.* Worldwide, it has been estimated that up to 645,000 respiratory deaths are associated with influenza annually.

Epidemics remain somewhat unpredictable with regard to the timing of onset and the severity of illness, but there are certain factors that may influence them. For example, epidemics are more likely to have originated in countries of the eastern or southern hemisphere, later spreading to Europe and North America. Epidemics may even be aided by the crowding of people during the cold weather in winter months. During a typical influenza epidemic, an estimated 10–20 percent of the population may become infected; however, in certain populations, it can reach 40–50 percent. The seasonality of the influenza virus is influenced by the humidity, and recent studies suggest that absolute humidity affects influenza virus transmission and survival more than relative humidity. Thus, influenza is less likely to be spread in hot, humid months in temperate climates, where epidemics tend to occur almost exclusively in winter months (October to April in the northern hemisphere compared to May to September in the southern hemisphere). In the tropics, influenza can be seen year round. Summertime epidemics of influenza can be sparked in contained, air-conditioned spaces, however; epidemics have occurred on cruise ships, barges, and nursing homes during the summer months in both the northern and southern hemispheres.

In most epidemics, a single strain of influenza will dominate. Influenza A epidemics typically begin rather abruptly and then peak over a two- to three-week period; they can last for two to three months in total. Usually, children are the first to suffer during epidemics, and then increases in adult infections soon follow. Eventually, influenza A epidemics often cause considerable absenteeism from school and work. Influenza B epidemics are generally less extensive and are associated with milder disease than those caused by influenza A. Often, the influenza B cases are reported in schools, military camps, chronic-care facilities, and nursing homes. On occasion, two different strains of influenza may circulate simultaneously. In addition, epidemics of influenza may occur during outbreaks of other respiratory viruses, such as adenovirus or respiratory syncytial virus. In some years, the end of an influenza epidemic is characterized by a brief spike in cases caused by an entirely new strain of flu. This is known as a herald wave, and it gives scientists a clue as to the likely dominant strain of the flu for the next season.

Pandemics

For an outbreak of influenza to eventually be labeled a pandemic, several conditions must be satisfied: (a) after arising in a specific geographical area, the outbreak of infection must spread globally; (b) there must be a high percentage of individuals who become infected, which then results in an increased death rate; and (c) the infection must be caused by a new influenza A strain that is not related to the viruses that circulated immediately before and did not arise via mutation from the preceding viruses. Influenza pandemics have recurred at somewhat irregular intervals since at least the ninth century, yet the signs and symptoms of influenza exhibited by those infected during pandemics haven't changed markedly over those centuries.

Some other characteristics of influenza pandemics include the following:

- Very rapid spread of the virus with outbreaks happening at the same time throughout the globe
- Diagnosis of the disease outside of its usual season (including the summer months)
- High rates of infection in all age groups with an increased risk for complications and death in healthy young adults who would not generally be affected by seasonal influenza

- More severe symptoms in infected people
- High likelihood of increased death rates
- Multiple waves of disease immediately before and after the main influenza outbreak

There are ongoing arguments in the medical and historical literature regarding the number of pandemics that have actually occurred as a result of influenza. Most references agree that there have been at least three major pandemics in the twentieth century. Many scientists believe that we don't currently have the tools to prevent the emergence of a future influenza pandemic, as the influenza viruses of the future are already mutating and evolving within wild waterfowl and other animals. Studying the details and understanding the historical, medical, and societal implications of past pandemics is necessary if preparation for a future pandemic is to be adequate. Further information on previous influenza pandemics can be found in chapter 2, while issues related to the possibility of a future influenza pandemic are discussed in chapters 9 and 10.

2

The History of Influenza

In a way, the history of influenza is akin to the history of humankind. Documentation of episodic illnesses that are now thought to be attributable to the influenza virus has been found dating back to 412 BCE. Outcomes of military battles, holy crusades, and world wars have been influenced by outbreaks, epidemics, and pandemics due to influenza. The research that led to the discovery of the influenza virus has contributed greatly to scientific confirmation of the germ theory. Governmental policies, fiscal decisions, and political outcomes have been directly linked to consequences of influenza. And still, the influenza virus and the illness it causes continue to influence history as it recurs season after season.

OUR UNDERSTANDING OF INFLUENZA

Hippocrates (460–375 BCE), the Greek physician and teacher known as the "Father of Medicine," believed, unlike many in his time, that diseases were not due to the influences of the gods, but rather were the result of natural causes. Other Greek physicians and philosophers also attempted to find specific causes to explain both mental and physical ailments. The elemental theory, as put forward by Empedocles (495–435 BCE), proposed that everything was composed of four elements (water, earth, air, and fire) and that these elements were moved by two opposing forces (love and strife). Disharmony of the elements, under the mixing and separating influences of the forces, was thought to result in physical ailments. Aristotle (384–322 BCE) further refined the elemental theory and began to associate it with certain temperaments, or personality traits. This eventually evolved into an even more advanced ill humor theory, which has been credited to Galen (AD 129–216). He believed that the four classic elements entered the body through food, drink, and the atmosphere; in the body, the elements were converted in specific organs to four fluids or humors: water to phlegm, earth to black bile, air to blood, and fire to yellow bile. Physical qualities were associated with each element and its corresponding humor. For example, the cold and wet months of winter were thought to contribute to production of phlegm, leading to cough and lung problems. The heat and dryness of summer, in contrast, shifted the humoral balance to yellow bile, leading to digestive diseases such as diarrhea. In addition to the physical characteristics, each humor was also thought to be associated with a particular temperament: black bile was associated with melancholic tendencies, while phlegm, blood, and yellow bile were linked to phlegmatic, sanguine, and choleric responses. A balance of these humors was thought to be necessary for good physical and mental health, and all sorts of practices (mostly unsuccessful) were used to try and keep the humors in harmony.

Despite the early Hippocratic teachings that suggested the existence of a natural disease process and a corresponding natural cure, these early theories of sickness were often influenced by the belief in various gods. For instance, Christians believed that groups of people who became ill with similar symptoms must have incited God's wrath because they had strayed from the presumed path of righteousness. Another religious emphasis was the association of disease and the "unclean." From the Middle Ages all the way into the mid-1800s, the miasma theory was a dominant belief. The miasma theory postulated that the air could become infested with a contagious influence when combined with the decomposing organic matter from the earth. The resulting vapor, or miasma, was thought to be the cause of diseases such as plague and cholera. Another theory that existed in the 1800s was based on the belief that there could be a sudden development of disease within the body. The blood generation theory supposed that a spontaneous chemical process in the blood made people sick.

It wasn't until the late 1800s that the germ theory was formulated. Louis Pasteur was a French scientist who was instrumental in providing evidence that germs existed, even if they couldn't be seen by the naked eye. Eventually, the germ theory was further refined by Robert Koch (1843–1910), a German physician and microbiologist. Koch took tissue samples from farm animals that were sick with a bacterial disease called anthrax and inoculated the samples into healthy mice, which then became ill and died from the same disease. In 1884, he outlined a set of criteria that established a link between an infectious agent and a specific disease process; Koch's postulates were further refined in 1890 and are as follows:

1. The infectious agent must be found in every case of the disease and in such a relationship to the damaged tissue so as to explain the damage.
2. The infectious agent must be isolated from a diseased organism and grown in pure culture outside of the body of its host.
3. The cultured agent, when introduced into a healthy animal, must produce a disease that is identical in its characteristics to the naturally occurring disease.
4. The microorganism must be able to be isolated from the inoculated, diseased experimental host and proven identical to the original infecting agent.

As the germ theory was becoming more widely accepted and further research was resulting in identification of pathogens as the agents responsible for many different diseases, scientists were eagerly looking for the cause of influenza. Indeed, for many years, it was thought that the illness known as the flu was caused by bacteria. Koch had an assistant, a German physician and bacteriologist named Richard Friedrich Johannes Pfeiffer (1858–1945). In 1892, Pfeiffer collected samples of mucus from sick patients who were thought to be suffering with the flu, and from these specimens, he was able to identify a small, rod-shaped bacterium. He called this organism *Bacillus influenzae*, but it became more commonly known as Pfeiffer's bacillus. Based on his findings, Pfeiffer published a report claiming that his bacillus was the causative agent of influenza. This didn't seem particularly unreasonable at the time, in part because bacteria had already been shown to cause other infectious diseases such as cholera and bubonic plague.

Pfeiffer's theory that his bacillus was the cause of influenza was not seriously challenged until many years later. During subsequent outbreaks of the flu in various parts of the world, researchers collected samples of respiratory secretions from sick patients, but they could not always find evidence of Pfeiffer's bacillus. Then, in 1918, an outbreak of a flu-like illness occurred at Camp Lewis in Washington. Scientists at Camp Lewis took mucus samples from their sick soldiers. Although the illness of many soldiers clearly fit with influenza, only a few of these samples showed growth of Pfeiffer's bacillus; some samples even showed growth of other bacteria. It was concluded that the illness that afflicted the soldiers at Camp Lewis was not due to Pfeiffer's bacillus, and it was further suggested that influenza might not be caused by a single bacterium at all. Around the same time, other medical researchers, when performing autopsies, found that the lungs of influenza patients did not have the same findings as lungs of patients who died of bacterial respiratory illnesses. The suspicion for a possible viral agent as the cause of influenza could not be ignored, despite considerable disagreement among highly respected medical personnel for years to come.

In the 1920s, two scientists named Peter K. Olitsky (1886–1964) and Frederick L. Gates (1853–1929), revisited the filter technique described previously by Chamberland (see chapter 1 for details). Olitsky and Gates took nasal secretions from presumed influenza patients and passed the specimens through a porcelain filter. As before, the filters were designed to stop most bacteria, but they would allow other smaller particles to pass through. The infectious agent in the secretions from flu patients easily passed through the filters. Around the same time, a researcher at the Pasteur Institute in Paris named Charles Jules Henry Nicolle (1866–1936) and his colleagues filtered the respiratory secretions from a patient with influenza and then injected this material into the eyes and nose of two monkeys. The monkeys quickly developed a fever. Then, the researchers administered the filtrate to a human volunteer by injecting it under the skin. The volunteer quickly became ill with symptoms consistent with influenza. Meanwhile, in Japan, researchers were also performing experiments on humans. They tested a number of healthy volunteers with filtered specimens from flu victims. All of their patients who had been inoculated with sputum and blood from flu victims came down with the flu except those who had already experienced an illness consistent with flu in the recent past; however, none of their subjects inoculated with bacterial preparations became sick with flu. With these studies, a virus as cause of the flu became entirely plausible.

A decade after Olitsky and Gates' filter experiment, a young American doctor named Richard Shope (1901–1966) began to study influenza under the guidance of his mentor, Paul Lewis (1879–1929). In 1929, a highly contagious respiratory illness was found to be spreading quickly through the swine on Iowa pig farms. A similar occurrence had been documented in swine in 1918, and to a smaller extent in the fall months of other years. Millions of pigs became ill with fever, runny noses, watery eyes, and respiratory symptoms; many pigs died. Because of the clinical similarities to the human illness, the disease was called swine flu. It occurred to Shope and Lewis that the agent that caused human influenza in 1918 might now be living in the pig population. Using Koch's postulates as a basis for experimentation, they first found a bacterium in the respiratory secretions taken from infected pigs and inoculated it into the noses of healthy pigs. Although the very first inoculated pig became ill, none of the other pigs tested thereafter became sick. Shope and Lewis concluded that the bacterium could *not* be the agent responsible for swine influenza. Remembering the filter technique performed by Olitsky and Gates, Shope decided to look for a virus. Mucus was collected from sick pigs and then filtered. The collected filtrate was inoculated into the noses of healthy pigs. These pigs became sick with a mild flu-like illness. Then, Shope took both the filtrate and the original bacterium and mixed them together. When this mixture was injected into healthy pigs, the swine became more severely ill with a full-blown influenza syndrome, including pneumonia. Shope concluded that the infectious agent causing swine influenza was in the filtered specimen (and thus more likely to be a virus) and that there might be a secondary infection in some pigs that was caused by the bacteria. By 1931, Shope had proven that the virus causing swine flu and the virus causing human flu were related but not identical.

As Shope was reaching his conclusions, a scientist in the United Kingdom named Christopher H. Andrewes (1896–1988) was also studying influenza. In 1933, an epidemic of influenza was identified in London and the surrounding area. Using Shope's techniques, Andrewes and his colleagues Wilson Smith (1897–1965) and Patrick Laidlaw (1881–1940) took filtered washings from sick patients and inoculated them into two ferrets. (Ferrets were thought to be good animals to use when studying influenza because they were susceptible to the disease and seemed to exist well in cages; unfortunately, though, they also could deliver a nasty bite. Luckily, over time, it was discovered that mice could be infected with the influenza virus and that they were much easier to study, and less likely to bite, than the ferrets.) Once inoculated with the filtered washings from the flu patients, the ferrets developed high fever, runny noses, and sneezing. These studies were repeated in a special facility in England, where the ferrets lived in complete isolation (this ensured that the ferrets were not contracting the flu naturally); the results were exactly the same. When Wilson Smith became ill with influenza after a sick ferret sneezed in his face, Andrewes isolated the viral strain and called it "WS." This strain was then used to inoculate future ferrets (and it is still available in the laboratory setting today). Andrewes, Smith, and Laidlaw were able to conclude that a virus was present in the filtered secretions from humans who were sick with flu, which could then be transmitted from humans to ferrets, from ferrets to humans (like in the case of the WS strain), and from ferret to ferret.

With the greater understanding of the influenza virus accomplished by experiments on pigs, ferrets, and mice, Shope and Andrewes were ready to turn their attention more fully to humans. They recruited volunteers of all ages in both the United States and England and collected blood samples from all subjects. They found that people who had survived the flu in 1918 had antibodies that blocked infection from Shope's swine flu virus. However, volunteers who had been born after 1918 didn't have these same protective antibodies. Other researchers then began to collect data in the field: patients who had been sick during various outbreaks of the flu were routinely tested, and all were found to have the same virus, which ultimately became known as influenza A. It is this viral strain that has the greatest impact on human disease and has been implicated in the major flu pandemics in history.

In 1935, Smith and Sir Frank Macfarlane Burnet (1899–1985) discovered that the flu virus could be grown in culture by using embryonated hens' eggs. The next year, the first neutralized antibodies generated by infection from the human influenza virus were isolated. Over the next half a decade, many more important developments took place in influenza research, including the demonstration that an inactivated version of the influenza virus could result in an antibody response in humans and that purification of the influenza virus by means of high-speed centrifugation could be accomplished.

In 1942, some years after the research by Shope and Andrewes confirmed the identification of influenza A, a second, but distinct, strain was found; this was called influenza B. Influenza B is primarily a disease of humans, although reports of infection in seals have been published. Influenza B has been responsible for seasonal outbreaks and epidemics of flu in humans. A third strain was not identified until almost 1950, and this was named influenza C; it tends to cause mild disease and is not of much significance to people. More recently, a new genus, called influenza D virus, was discovered in pigs and cattle in the United States and Europe.

MAJOR INFLUENZA EPIDEMICS AND PANDEMICS

As noted in the introduction to this book, as early as 412 BCE, Hippocrates described an outbreak of a clinical syndrome that was suggestive of influenza. In 212 BCE, a historian named Titus Livius authored the *History of Rome* and noted that the Roman Army had been "visited by pestilence, a calamity almost heavy enough to turn them from all thoughts of war"; this outbreak has been suggested to be due to influenza. In 855, an epidemic thought possibly due to flu started in Central Asia and spread across Persia. Twenty-one years later, a flu epidemic spread across Europe and slowed Charlemagne's conquest as the illness claimed the lives of much of his army. In the years 1173 and 1500, two influenza outbreaks were described, though with little detail. Large outbreaks and epidemics of influenza were then noted in 1510 (described in detailed and reliable fashion as the virus spread from Africa to Europe) and again in 1557, when concern for worldwide spread was noted. In 1580, the first definite and well-documented pandemic due to influenza occurred. It originated in

Asia and Russia during the summer months, spread to Africa, then Europe, and eventually landed in the Americas. The pandemic of 1580 was known to have caused the death of over 8,000 people in Rome, while in Spain, it decimated the populations of entire cities. Over the centuries, further major epidemics and pandemics were described. From 1404 to the middle of the nineteenth century, 31 influenza epidemics were recorded, including eight large-scale pandemics. Some of the most notable outbreaks occurred in 1729 (originating in Russia and spreading throughout Europe within six months), in 1781 (a pandemic spreading from China to Russia, Europe, and North America), in 1830 (a pandemic that spread from China to India, the Philippines, Indonesia, Russia, Europe, and North America), in 1847, in 1857, and in 1898 (a pandemic that spread from Europe to India, Australia, and North and South America).

Spanish Flu: The Pandemic of 1918

It is difficult to describe the dramatic and devastating medical event that is now known as the influenza pandemic of 1918. Author J. I. Waring labeled it as "the greatest medical holocaust in history." In the United States alone, one of every four people suffered from some effect of the flu, and more than 500,000 deaths were recorded. One-third of the world's population was infected with the influenza virus and showed evidence of illness during this pandemic, and an estimated 20–50 million people died (although some suggest that this number may actually be closer to 100 million). This pandemic was responsible for more deaths than all of the major wars of the twentieth century combined.

The origin of the first wave of the 1918 pandemic is still not known. Some literature suggests that it may have originated in China, but other documentation describes several of the first outbreaks in the United States. A cook at Camp Fuston in Kansas named Albert Gitchel became ill with a fever, cough, and headache on March 4, 1918; he was one of the first established cases of influenza at the start of the pandemic. Within three weeks, 1,100 other soldiers had been hospitalized, and thousands more were sick. Regardless of its origin, the infection traveled unchecked, aided by the other notable event happening at that time in history: World War I. The United States entered the war in April 1917, and in March 1918, nearly 100,000 American troops were sent to Europe; the following month, almost 120,000 more made the trip. An outbreak of typical seasonal springtime influenza had already begun in the United States before the troops were deployed, and unfortunately, soldiers who were suffering from flu were among those traveling across the globe. When American troops arrived at the military depot in Bordeaux, so did influenza: three-quarters of the French troops fell ill. From France, the virus then spread to the British Expeditionary Force (more than half of the British troops became sick) and to other European soldiers. By late April and May, the infection had reached Italy, Spain, and Germany. In June, influenza reached England, Scotland, and Wales. It then struck Portugal and then moved on to Greece. From there, it hit Murmansk and Russia. And then it quickly traveled to North Africa, India, China, New Zealand, and the Philippines. In most every country, the infection spread for several weeks and then faded sharply. Only an occasional outbreak was noted during the summer months of 1918 in the United States. As the war continued, healthy American soldiers continued to ship out to Europe. During June, July, and August 1918, more than half a million troops made the trip. Despite feeling well as they left the States, the soldiers arrived in Europe just as a second wave of influenza was being recognized. The virus followed the travel of the troops throughout Europe and again across the globe. By January 1919, the pandemic had reached Australia.

It began to be apparent that the second wave of infection was impressively severe and that the death rate was high. In addition to targeting the very young and old as influenza was already known to do, it was also attacking young, healthy adults (particularly those between 20 and 29 years of age) at a rate that had never been seen before. In many nations, a third wave occurred in early 1919. In India, an estimated 20 million people perished. Cape Town reported that 4 percent of their population died of influenza in the first four weeks of the outbreak there. Ten percent of the population died in Chiapas, Mexico. In Brazil, attack rates reached 33 percent; in Buenos Aires, Argentina, they exceeded 50 percent. In Japan, the virus made more than one-third of the entire population sick. Both Russia and Iran lost 7 percent of their population to the flu. In the United States, over one-quarter of the population suffered from influenza during the pandemic. In all of North America, 600,000 people died, including 25 percent of the population in Samoa and Alaska. Deaths of young adults in the United States were so significant during the pandemic that the life expectancy dropped by more than 10 years in 1918.

Though the pandemic did not start in Spain, it still became known as the Spanish flu. This was due to the fact that Spain was a neutral country in the war and did not have governmental censorship of its press like France, Germany, and England. The Spanish newspapers honestly reported the presence of influenza (including the illness of King Alphonse XIII), and they were one of the few countries to report the effect of the virus on their troops and their civilians. The strain that caused the 1918 pandemic was H1N1 with genes of avian origin. The impact of this novel virus is not limited only to 1918, as descendants of the H1N1 virus still circulate today.

Asian Flu: The Pandemic of 1957–1958

After the pandemic of 1918, influenza continued to cause seasonal regional epidemics in a more usual pattern. But in 1957, a new viral strain emerged. The Asian flu pandemic started in the Yunan Province of China in February of that year. After causing many to become ill in China, it spread to Singapore, Hong Kong, Taiwan, and Japan. Infection then moved to India, Australia, and Indonesia in May; to Pakistan, Europe, North America, and the Middle East in June; to South Africa, South America, New Zealand, and the Pacific Islands in July; and to Central, West, and East Africa, Eastern Europe, and the Caribbean in August.

Interestingly, a particular route of transmission for the Asian flu strain was traced to a large conference held in Iowa that year. Eighteen hundred young adults from 43 different states and several foreign countries attended the conference, and 200 of them became ill with the flu. Suffering from their illness, these young adults then returned to their homes, taking the virus with them. Another route of transmission was identified from Russia to Scandinavia and Eastern Europe; otherwise, though, the infection seemed to have spread by sea travel. Within six months, the infection was worldwide, and more than a million people died during the pandemic (including 116,000 in the United States).

This pandemic was the first that occurred in the modern age of viral research, and this virus was available for laboratory investigation. The strain was identified as H2N2, a subtype that had never before been seen in the human population; both the HA and NA antigens were unlike any previously found in humans. This new virus had impressive NA activity, and it was more stable than earlier influenza strains. It also differed from other viruses in terms of neutralization with antibodies or HA inhibition. It was shown that the virus alone, even without secondary bacterial infection, was able to kill those who became infected.

A second wave of flu occurred in early 1958, with regions in Europe, North American, Russia, and Japan being affected. In some countries, the second wave was more severe than the first. In total, the pandemic affected 40–50 percent of the world's population, with 25–30 percent showing signs or symptoms of the disease. One out of every four thousand people was estimated to have died from the flu, and most deaths occurred in the very young and the very old.

Because this viral strain was unfamiliar to most of the human population, it was the first pandemic in which a vaccine response could be observed. Studies later showed that more vaccines were required to initiate an initial antibody response than had been observed previously and that divided doses were more beneficial than a single injection.

Further surveillance in the post-pandemic period shows that the H2N2 virus survived only 11 years; after that point, a new subtype (H3N2) emerged.

Hong Kong Flu: The Pandemic of 1968–1969

The Hong Kong flu pandemic killed thousands of people worldwide (estimates suggest 1 million deaths), including 100,000 people in the United States, mostly in people 65 years of age and older. It began in Hong Kong in the summer months, traveled to Vietnam and Singapore, and eventually on to India, the Philippines, Australia, and Europe. It arrived in the United States in September, but then peaked in December of 1968 and January of 1969. Initially, illness occurred in the absence of increased death rates. However, additional waves in 1969 and 1970 were deadlier (especially in the United States) and included cases in Japan, Africa, and South America.

The strain that was responsible for the Hong Kong pandemic was identified as H3N2. It was discovered that the N2 antigen was similar to its precursor (H2N2), but the HA antigen differed and was presumed to be avian in origin. These distinctions were thought to explain the lower death rates than in previous pandemics, as some people may have had partial immunity from past exposure to the 1957 Asian flu strain. Other factors that may have influenced the death rate included improved access to medical care than in the past and the increased availability of antibiotics to help treat secondary bacterial infection.

Interestingly, the descendants of this H3N2 virus are still the major and most troublesome seasonal influenza A viruses in circulation in humans today.

Swine Flu: The Epidemic of 1976

In January 1976, a young army private named David Lewis began to feel ill while stationed at Fort Dix, a training center in New Jersey. Though his medical officer assigned him to his quarters, Lewis joined his platoon for an all-night hike in the winter weather. After managing to march for a period of time despite his illness, Lewis eventually collapsed, and within hours, he was dead with the diagnosis of influenza. By the end of the month, at least 300 recruits at Fort Dix were sick with influenza. A team of scientists at the New Jersey State Health Department Laboratory were able to test many of the soldiers' respiratory specimens (and they tested a sample from Lewis on autopsy, too). They found that the Fort Dix patients had antibodies that worked against the swine flu that had initially been isolated by Shope. It was already known that people who survived the Spanish flu in 1918 also had these antibodies, so it was thought that the Fort Dix flu virus might be the same as, or at least similar to, the virus that had caused the earlier pandemic.

The Centers for Disease Control and Prevention (CDC) in Atlanta was contacted, and it quickly repeated and confirmed the results. The infecting strain was identified as H1N1, which was different than the H3N2 strain that was already causing seasonal influenza elsewhere in the United States that year (some of the soldiers at Fort Dix also had evidence of this strain of flu). Concerned about an evolving pandemic that could mimic that which occurred in 1918, the U.S. government reacted quickly. In March, a group of scientists gathered at the White House and came to the agreement that mass vaccination was necessary. In August, President Gerald R. Ford authorized the National Swine Flu Immunization Program of 1976 with $135 million dedicated to the production and administration of a vaccine. Vaccination for the swine flu officially began on October 1, and within 10 months, roughly 25 percent of the U.S. population was vaccinated. As happens in politics, some members of Congress added on almost $2 billion of social service spending and environmental protection funds to the president's immunization act. Contributing to this financial burden was the position of the pharmaceutical manufacturers, who told President Ford that the government would have to assume all liabilities for possible ill effects from the vaccines.

Progress on the vaccination campaign stalled when a report of three elderly patients' deaths within days of receiving the vaccine surfaced. Although these deaths were later shown to be coincidental and not in any way related to the vaccine, the public's perception about the swine flu vaccine had already been affected. In November, a man in Minnesota was diagnosed with a form of paralysis after receiving the vaccination; this was quickly followed by more than 1,100 reports of similar illnesses, although only half of these were in people who had actually received the swine flu vaccine. This resulted in a legal nightmare with more than 4,000 claims filed with the U.S. attorney general's office on behalf of clients who allegedly suffered ailments because of the swine flu vaccine; these claims totaled over $3.2 billion. Over the next 15 years, the U.S. government continued to battle legal claims (some were settled costing more than $37 million, some ended up in the courtroom costing $17 million, and some were lost in litigation costing more than $30 million).

Overall, the Swine Flu Immunization Program of 1976 was both a financial and a political disaster. The American government spent billions of dollars on the vaccine campaign and its subsequent legal claims, but swine flu actually remained relatively rare overall in 1976, even among people who didn't receive the vaccine. No other deaths occurred at Fort Dix, and most of the infections that year were due to the usual seasonal influenza strain (H3N2). Perhaps not surprisingly, President Ford lost his reelection bid in November 1976.

Russian Flu: The Epidemic of 1977

In November 1977, a new strain of H1N1 was identified in Russia, and it looked to be similar to the virus that had been seen before 1957. Later, it was found to have been reported in northeastern China in May of that year, but the label of Russian flu (or Red Influenza or Red Flu) had already taken hold. The virus spread rapidly, and it was almost entirely restricted to persons under 25 years of age. In general, though, the infection itself seemed to be mild in severity, and the symptoms were as would be expected for typical influenza. The age distribution was thought to be due to the absence of exposure to the H1N1 virus in humans born after 1957 and the dominance beyond that year of the H2N2 subtype, followed by the H3N2 strain. Later studies of this H1N1 strain showed that both the HA and NA antigens were very similar to circulating viral strains from the 1950s.

Swine Flu: The Pandemic of 2009

In the spring of 2009, a novel H1N1 flu strain emerged. It was first detected in the United States, though the first outbreak was described in Mexico; regardless, it spread rapidly across the globe. By June 2009, the World Health Organization (WHO) declared that a global pandemic was underway. This new virus was made up of the genetic elements from four different strains of influenza (North American swine, North American avian, human, and Asia/European swine), and it was designated as influenza A (H1N1)pdm09. This virus had never before been seen in either people or animals. As it was first being isolated, it was thought that people were being exposed to the virus through contact with pigs; however, as the pandemic unfolded, it became clear that the virus was primarily spreading from person to person.

Although young people had no existing immunity to the (H1N1)pdm09 virus, about one-third of people over 60 years of age had antibodies against this virus thought likely to be the result of exposure to an older H1N1 virus earlier in their lives. Given the novelty of this viral strain, the seasonal flu vaccines in 2009 offered little protection against infection due to (H1N1)pdm09. A pandemic vaccine was produced but was not available in large quantities until November 2009; the peak of illness during a second wave had already come and gone in the United States by then.

Luckily, the virus didn't seem to have any of the markers that were thought to be associated with increased risk of severe disease or high death rates like previous pandemic viral strains. Despite this, though, (H1N1) pdm09 killed an estimated half-million people worldwide, and 80 percent of these deaths occurred in people younger than 65 years of age. In the United States alone, there were 60 million reported cases of infection, more than 274,000 hospitalizations, and over 12,000 deaths. On August 10, 2010, the pandemic was declared over. The (H1N1)pdm09 virus, more commonly known as pH1N1, continues to circulate as a seasonal flu virus to this day.

Newer Influenza Strains

Every year, usual seasonal flu viruses like H3N2 circulate among the human population. However, the influenza virus is decidedly skillful in its ability to mutate, and it is the concern about emergence of a new viral strain that prompts aggressive vaccination campaigns and other strategies to prevent another major pandemic (or at least minimize the potential for catastrophic consequences should one occur). It took almost 40 years after the Spanish flu of 1918 for the next novel influenza virus to emerge; it took another 10 years after that for the next one. But between 2011 and 2015, seven new strains were identified in humans, and they have appeared all over the world (in China, Egypt, United States, and Europe).

One of the newer influenza strains that has caused considerable concern is H5N1, which was responsible for a bird flu scare in 1997. This strain was first identified in Hong Kong, and it was thought to have spread from chickens at poultry farms and markets directly to humans. During the 12 months of 1997, it infected 18 people who had handled poultry. More than 60 percent of those infected suffered from severe pneumonia and over half required treatment in an intensive care unit; six of the infected people died. In response to the outbreak, the entire poultry population (more than 1 million chickens) in China was destroyed within three days. Despite this, the H5N1 strain continues to circulate among humans across the globe (though numbers are low) with an impressive lethality.

Other avian influenza viruses have been linked to human disease in more recent years, including H7N2 in the United States and the United Kingdom, H7N3 in Canada, H7N7 in the Netherlands, H7N9 in China, H9N2 in Hong Kong, H10N7 in Egypt, and H10N8 in China. Further discussion about the ability of the influenza virus to mutate and the discovery of novel influenza strains can be found in chapter 3.

ADVANCES IN INFLUENZA TREATMENT AND PREVENTION

Clearly, influenza is an impressive virus. It manages to evade human defenses to cause large numbers of infections year after year in seasonal outbreaks and epidemics. It mutates to form novel strains that result in worldwide pandemics. And it contributes to significant personal, societal, economic, and health care burdens across the globe. It is no surprise, then, that much of the focus of influenza research has been on treatment and prevention.

Historical Remedies

Before the germ theory was widely understood and accepted, ancient physicians and healers who believed in the elemental or ill humor theories tried various remedies to combat symptoms of infection: manipulations of the diet, ingestion of potions, use of substances designed to force a patient to vomit, and methods of draining blood (even using leeches). As the miasma theory was introduced, physicians proposed that patients might benefit from aggressive antiseptic cleansing of their bodies, that people should not shake hands with one another, and that gauze masks be worn whenever people ventured outdoors. In the late 1880s, people in England carried carbolic smoke balls (a rubber ball that, when squeezed, emitted a puff of carbolic acid that would be inhaled). One tribal technique required that the still-warm and bleeding skin of a sheep or lamb be placed on the chest. During the Spanish flu pandemic, people wore necklaces of garlic or camphor balls, wrapped peeled garlic cloves in muslin and pinned them to their underwear, rubbed wormwood or steamed horse manure on their chests, injected eucalyptus oil rectally, placed onions around the house, and drank pine tar (a combination of charcoal and pine that was used as a wood sealant). In more contemporary times, over-the-counter cold and flu medications have been commonly used. Unfortunately, these supportive measures often offered little to no benefit, and occasionally, they could even be harmful.

Development of Vaccines

As early as 1000 BCE, a process known as variolation was described. This referred to a technique in which pus or scabs taken from active smallpox (a disease caused by a virus named variola) on one patient were rubbed into the skin of another. Although this technique did not always prevent smallpox infection, it did seem to reduce the death rate among people already infected. Edward Jenner (1749–1823), a physician in England, was intrigued by the success of variolation, particularly when he realized that milkmaids who had been infected with cowpox (a disease caused by a virus related to variola) did not seem to become infected with smallpox. Bravely, Jenner injected cowpox into a healthy young boy and then exposed the boy to smallpox; the boy did not show any lesions of smallpox. Jenner called this process vaccination (taken from the Latin term *vacca*, meaning cow). Though it took time for the medical community (and the general public) to accept vaccination as a legitimate technique, it eventually led to eradication of the disease known as smallpox.

The general concept of vaccination is quite simple, actually. In response to exposure to an infectious agent, the human body produces proteins called antibodies; the purpose of antibodies is to neutralize or destroy germs. Antibodies are disease-specific, meaning that the influenza antibodies produced in response to infection with the influenza virus will only work against the flu. So, by administering low levels of an infectious agent (or an agent so similar to the germ that it can "trick" the body) via a vaccine, antibodies can be produced for future protection against the infection; this protected state is known as immunity. Because of the influenza virus's ability to mutate, though, the issues that surround successful influenza vaccination are more complicated than those involving other infectious agents such as polio or measles. This difficulty explains why the influenza vaccine doesn't grant lifelong immunity and must be administered annually; this concept will be discussed further in chapter 8.

In addition to his contributions to germ theory, Louis Pasteur made the first known attempt to vaccinate humans with a live virus (rabies, actually), which was attenuated (or weakened) so that it was less virulent and unable to cause harmful infection yet was still able to produce an antibody reaction. In 1936, following in Pasteur's footsteps, a scientist in the Soviet Union injected an attenuated influenza virus into human subjects; though they developed a slight fever, they were found to be protected against reinfection. The following year, Smith, Andrewes, and Charles Stuart-Harris (1909–1996) conducted a study among the military forces in England using an inactivated influenza strain isolated from a mouse lung in a subcutaneous vaccine.

In the next few years, the need for an influenza vaccine intensified along with the threat of another world war. Scientists first had to figure out how to grow and maintain the virus in a way that didn't include passing it from one animal to another as had been done for years in the lab. Though this approach obviously worked well with ferrets and mice, the process was slow and often required three weeks from start to finish. In 1940, the virus was successfully grown on the embryos of chicken eggs; this virus grew quickly and in high concentrations, too. Once it was determined that the virus could be isolated by inoculation into the amniotic cavity of the egg, animal use became unnecessary. By 1942, there were three additional techniques that helped in vaccine production: centrifugation, freezing and thawing the allantoic fluid in the embryonated chicken eggs, and absorption of the virus into red cells at low temperature and their removal at higher temperature. In the United States, the military was key in moving vaccine research and production forward. In 1941, the army created a Commission on Influenza and Vaccine Development; this commission (later known as the Armed Forces Epidemiological Board) eventually led to a program to control influenza during World War II and was a focus of American influenza research for 20 years.

The first influenza vaccine was a whole virus, inactivated, monovalent preparation—this means that it contained only one subtype of the influenza A virus and that it had been attenuated for administration. In December 1942, large influenza vaccine studies were begun; these were successful in proving that the inactivated influenza virus vaccines were effective protection against flu epidemics. During ongoing vaccine studies between 1942 and 1945, however, a phenomenon of "influenza mismatch" was identified: the virus contained in the vaccine didn't match the circulating viral strain that was causing the seasonal epidemics. One reason for this was that there was a new strain of flu virus in circulation (influenza B); the other reason for this was the effect of major and minor mutations of the circulating influenza A viruses. With the aid of the Armed Forces Epidemiological Board, the development of an inactivated bivalent vaccine that could be delivered subcutaneously was accomplished; this type of vaccine contained two influenza viral strains: one type A and one type B. This vaccine was first tested and approved for military use in the United States. In 1946, the bivalent, inactivated vaccine was approved for civilian use. That same year, a new variant of influenza A appeared in Australia, followed by the identification of the new influenza A subtype known as H2N2, which caused the Asian flu pandemic; the next year, the U.S. Commission on Influenza recommended that H2N2 be included in subsequent vaccines.

In light of the "influenza mismatch" phenomenon, a system for the surveillance of circulating influenza viruses was necessary to help guide decisions about yearly vaccine production. In 1952, WHO created the Influenza Study Center, designed to monitor circulating viral strains in several countries; this has since been expanded. Each year, WHO determines which strains of influenza will make up the vaccination components based on results of this global surveillance, attempting to predict how the influenza virus has mutated over the last year and how the virus will spread in the northern and southern hemispheres (which can require different vaccines). Obviously, these predictions are exceedingly tricky, and influenza vaccine effectiveness can vary widely. According to the CDC, during the

2004–2005 influenza season, the vaccine effectiveness was estimated to be 10 percent; however, the vaccine effectiveness for the 2010–2011 influenza season was 60 percent.

Research continued as new inactivated compounds were tested for safety and efficacy during seasonal influenza epidemics. At the same time, the U.S. government passed the Vaccination Assistance Act of 1962; this encouraged extensive immunizations by allowing financial support for the vaccine programs of both state and local health departments. Two years later, the Advisory Committee on Immunization Practices was started with the specific task of providing the CDC with recommendations on vaccine use; it has continued to release vaccine recommendations to this day. During the 1960s, two new vaccine formulations were created: the split vaccine (which has an additional treatment step with detergent to break open the viral envelope and allow all the viral proteins and subviral elements to be exposed) and the subunit vaccine (which contains only purified and enriched HA and NA antigens). These new types of vaccines were proven to have decreased adverse reactions in children when compared to the whole virus vaccines, especially in the early years of life. The first flu vaccines were then licensed in Europe, and in the United States, it was recommended that individuals at major risk of complications from the flu undergo annual influenza vaccination. In 1968, the new viral strain H3N2 appeared (this strain was the cause of the Hong Kong flu pandemic), completely replacing the H2N2 strain in circulation.

By the 1970s, researchers had unveiled the first trivalent, or three-component, influenza vaccine, known as TIV; this vaccine contained two influenza A strains (H1N1 and H3N2) and one influenza B strain. Split vaccines were used during the Swine Flu pandemic, when the H1N1 subtype re-emerged. Though side effects to the split vaccines seemed to be decreased when compared to the earlier whole-virus vaccines, the split vaccines unfortunately showed less of an immune reaction in people who had never before been vaccinated against the flu; thus, two vaccine doses were needed to ensure effective protection in these "unprimed" individuals. By the late 1970s, the first subunit vaccine was able to be administered; these vaccines were also shown to have decreased immunogenicity.

Much of the focus on influenza vaccination continued to be on new techniques of immunization that might be better tolerated and provide a greater immune response. In 2003, the use of a live attenuated vaccine that was delivered intranasally was approved in the United States. This vaccine was determined appropriate for healthy, nonpregnant people between the ages of 5 and 49. In 2007, it was approved for younger children between the ages of two and five; this was a welcome alternative to vaccine injections for the pediatric population. That same year, the Food and Drug Administration (FDA) in the United States approved the first vaccination for humans against the avian influenza virus H5N1. In 2009, a new high-dose influenza vaccine was recommended for the elderly due to waning of immunity with aging; this vaccine consisted of a new formulation that contained a fourfold higher HA dose than the traditional TIV. This was followed in 2011 by the first FDA approval for an intradermal flu vaccine.

In 2012, the first quadrivalent vaccine was introduced; this split vaccine contained two influenza A strains and two influenza B strains. The presence of the additional influenza B strain was meant to further reduce the possibility of a mismatch between the circulating influenza viruses and the vaccine composition, while still offering people the same safety and successful immune response. The following year, a recombinant trivalent influenza vaccine was approved by the FDA for people aged 18–49 years. This was the first trivalent influenza vaccine made using recombinant DNA technology, and it was licensed as a spray formulation.

The surveillance of influenza activity continues in labs across the globe, sponsored by the WHO, which then releases a recommended vaccine formula for each region of the world. In the United States, both the CDC and the FDA collaborate to ensure the safety, effectiveness, and security of vaccines. The Influenza Branch of the CDC is in charge of influenza surveillance in the United States, while the Immunization Safety Office leads most of the agency's vaccine safety and research monitoring. Now, much of the research in influenza prevention has shifted toward the development of a universal vaccine. Back in 2008, a specific human antibody that protects against a broad spectrum of influenza viruses was discovered, and with this discovery, researchers realized that humans were capable of producing antibodies against a part of the influenza virus that doesn't change from season to season. More information about universal vaccination research can be found in chapter 10.

Availability of Medications

As research allowed identification of the influenza virus and its unique characteristics, scientists began to study ways to inhibit the virus, hoping to either prevent infection or offer treatment against the infection should it occur. Historically, there have been two main categories of influenza antiviral medications: M2 inhibitors and neuraminidase inhibitors; however, just recently, a new class of medications known as endonuclease inhibitors has been approved for use.

M2 inhibitors essentially prevent shedding of influenza's viral envelope, which inhibits entry of the viral particle into the human host cell. The first available drug in this class, amantadine, was released in the 1960s; rimantadine, a derivative of amantadine, followed in the early 1990s. These two medications are only active against influenza A, and unfortunately, due to increased resistance, this class of medications is no longer recommended for influenza treatment or prevention.

The antiviral medications known as neuraminidase inhibitors offer benefit by rendering NA useless so that the influenza virus remains connected to its host cell and is unable to travel to other cells or to a new host. In 1999, two neuraminidase inhibitors were approved by the FDA for the treatment of influenza A and B: oseltamivir and zanamivir. A newer agent in this class, peramivir, was approved for use in 2014. Unlike the earlier medications in this class, peramivir can be given intravenously and only requires one dose; this allows antiviral treatment to be administered to people who cannot swallow or digest pills. Both oseltamivir and zanamivir can be used as treatment or prevention against the flu; peramivir is only recommended as a treatment alternative.

The newer endonuclease inhibitors block viral proliferation. Baloxavir is an anti-influenza medication in this class that was just approved for treatment in 2018; it works for both influenza A and B. It is not currently recommended for prevention. More detailed information about antiviral medications can be found in chapter 5 (treatment) and chapter 8 (prevention).

3

Causes and Risk Factors

When a virulent pathogen comes in contact with a desired host, infection can occur. In the case of the influenza virus, the epithelial cells of the human respiratory tract are its goal. Droplets of respiratory secretions, laden with viral particles, are sent into the air by sneezing, coughing, or even talking. They don't remain suspended in the air for long and travel less than one meter in most circumstances. These droplets can then enter the respiratory tract of a new host (either directly or by hands that have come in contact with surfaces contaminated with droplets), causing yet another person to become infected with influenza.

WHY DO HUMANS GET THE FLU?

Once the influenza virus has been taken in by the respiratory epithelial cells of a host, replication of more viral particles begins, allowing new virions to be released to infect adjacent cells. After infection, most people will have an interval of time during which no symptoms are felt, known as the incubation period. Although the length of the incubation period varies for each germ, it typically lasts just a few days with influenza (and in some lucky patients, little or no symptoms are ever appreciated, even beyond the incubation period). Eventually, the infected cells die, which triggers the immune system to produce antibodies and other protective substances.

Given that the immune response to infection with influenza is vigorous, why don't humans develop lifelong immunity to the virus? And why do seasonal influenza epidemics continue to happen every year across the globe?

Influenza Antigenic Drift and Shift

Interestingly, the answer to these questions is related to one particular characteristic of the influenza virus: it is decidedly skillful in its ability to alter its surface proteins. As has been discussed previously, the glycoprotein spikes on the surface of the influenza virus, hemagglutinin (HA) and neuraminidase (NA), allow the viral particle to enter a host's respiratory epithelial cells in order to undergo protein synthesis and, ultimately, to succeed in producing more influenza viral particles through replication. However, the genes that encode for the HA and NA proteins are found in an RNA, rather than DNA, backbone. Though this might seem to be a rather subtle distinction, it is important when considering the influenza virus's ability to change through mutation. DNA-based viruses have a special proofreading enzyme that carefully monitors the process of copying a strand of DNA, catching and correcting any mistakes made during replication. Unfortunately, RNA-based viruses like influenza don't have a proofreader. During replication of the virus, mistakes occur, particularly with regard to the HA and NA proteins. The mistakes are often at points on the HA and NA proteins that are antigenic, or capable of being recognized by antibodies as a binding site. The influenza virus is able to mutate so quickly that 99 percent of the new viral particles produced in a host cell are defective. Most of the mutations cause defects that are severe enough to either destroy the new virion completely or stop it from infecting a new cell. Other mutations, though, allow the new viral particle to adapt and continue with further replication, potentially producing a more dangerous infectious agent because prior antibodies against the flu won't work with the altered HA and NA antigen sites.

Small genetic mutations, known as antigenic drift, usually produce viruses that are closely related to one another. Luckily, in these circumstances, the antigenic sites are similar among the viral strains, and the human immune system may still be able to recognize them in order to respond appropriately if infection occurs. However, small mutations can accumulate over time and eventually result in a virus that is quite antigenically different from previous strains. As antigenic drift continues, the number of protective antibodies that were produced during infection in earlier years declines. Humans become less and less able to defend themselves against a constantly mutating virus because their old antibodies may not recognize a newly changed viral strain or the old antibodies may not work as well as they did in the past. Antigenic drift explains, then, the repeated pattern of influenza outbreaks and epidemics for centuries on end. It also explains why we can get sick with flu again and again, year after year. Scientists and public health experts monitor the antigenic drift of influenza carefully, and the influenza vaccine produced each year attempts to take into consideration the possible mutations that might have influenced the next season's viral strains.

Interestingly, though, the influenza strains that have caused pandemic flu in the past did not arise by the small mutations of existing strains due to antigenic drift. Instead, they have been found to be caused by entirely new viral strains. Thus, the origin of these novel viruses remains the focus of much research as efforts to reduce risk and consequence of a future pandemic are made. The most accepted theory suggests that pandemic viruses arise from a cross of animal and human strains with abrupt and drastic changes in the viral HA and NA structures; this phenomenon is known as antigenic shift. In this process, animal influenza viruses and human influenza viruses initiate a "combined infection" in a cell of a species in which they can both multiply. While replicating, the virus undergoes reassortment with genetic material from each strain. This theoretically allows infectivity in humans, but with the presence of animal glycoproteins to which the majority of the human population has never before been exposed (and thus has no antibodies or immune protection). If two different viruses infect a cell, an exchange of gene segments can easily take place and *hundreds* of different "offspring" are possible. The "offspring" viral particles, in turn, have the potential to infect many, many humans with no hope of immunity.

Influenza viruses mutate via antigenic drift all the time, but fortunately, antigenic shift happens only occasionally. Influenza A viruses undergo both kinds of changes; influenza B viruses change only by antigenic drift. The most recent antigenic shift occurred with the Swine Flu pandemic of 2009. The H1N1 virus that caused this pandemic had genes from North American pigs, Eurasian pigs, humans, and birds.

Significant Influenza Strains

In the United States, seasonal epidemics due to influenza A and B viruses occur each fall, winter, and spring; influenza C virus infections occur sporadically. Currently, the viruses that cause the seasonal epidemics in humans are influenza A/pH1N1 and influenza A/H3N2. While influenza B viruses are not classified into subtypes, they are broken down into lineages; the strains currently in circulation belong to either B/Yamagata or B/Victoria lineages.

Obviously, novel influenza A viruses that arise from antigenic shift (like the one that caused the Swine Flu in 2009) are a major cause for concern, as they have been the culprits in past influenza pandemics, and it is postulated that this phenomenon will cause a pandemic in the future, too. The viruses that have caused pandemics can then become recurrent seasonal strains. For example, the H1N1 virus that caused the 1918 Spanish influenza pandemic became a common flu strain, and the most recent version is known as pH1N1 due to its continued circulation beyond the pandemic of 2009.

Other significant influenza strains have been identified in recent years, and all are being monitored closely.

- H9N2 is an influenza strain that was known to be found in turkeys. In the 1990s, it was isolated in humans in China, and subsequent human infections have been reported from Egypt, Bangladesh, Pakistan, and Oman. Fortunately, thus far, human infections have mostly been mild with only one death.
- First discovered in 2003, a viral strain known as H5N1 has continued to cause concern. An avian virus, H5N1 has mostly infected people in Asia and northeast Africa, especially Egypt and Indonesia. In each of these areas, avoidance of poultry farms, bird markets, or other places where live poultry are raised, kept, or sold was recommended. There has been no evidence of person-to-person spread with this virus.
- A variant of the H3N2 virus known as H3N2v was noted to cause illness in 12 people in 2011. This was a strain that was already recognized as a cause of swine flu, but it subsequently became transmittable to humans. This strain continues to circulate, but it has caused limited cases of influenza in people.
- In 2013, an outbreak with H7N9 was identified in China. This viral strain was avian in origin, and it was thought that the affected people who became ill with H7N9 were exposed to infected poultry, especially at live bird markets. This particular strain did not appear to be transmittable between humans. However, this virus was particularly worrisome because of the high death rate among those infected.
- An avian influenza strain originating in China, labeled H10N8, has been described since 2014. This strain has been proven to be deadly to humans.
- In 2015, a highly pathogenic avian strain labeled HPAIH5 was identified. This was discovered both in wild, migratory birds (such as Canadian geese, Mallard ducks, and the Snowy owl) and domestic poultry, including chickens, turkeys, and ducks.
- An outbreak of canine influenza in Chicago was attributed to an H3N2 strain in 2015. This virus originated in horses, and from there, it easily spread to dogs. Luckily, this particular influenza strain has not been shown to be transmittable to humans.

WHO IS MOST LIKELY TO GET REALLY SICK FROM THE FLU?

Influenza A, B, and C viruses all cause infection of the human respiratory tract, but the symptoms can vary greatly. Some people who become infected with the flu have no symptoms at all, while others have infections that are much more complicated. Most people recover from the flu without any long-term ill effects, but some are considered to be at increased risk for severe, and potentially even fatal, influenza infection.

Children

Children under five years of age are particularly vulnerable to more complicated infections with influenza, particularly if they are younger than two years of age. It has been estimated that 15–42 percent of preschool and school-aged children become infected with influenza each year, and these infections are associated with an increased number of outpatient health care visits, increased rates of hospitalization, more absences from school for both the child and their siblings, and many missed workdays for parents. Very young children, or children with certain medical conditions, are particularly vulnerable. This includes children with chronic pulmonary diseases (such as asthma or cystic fibrosis), conditions that compromise respiratory function or ability to handle secretions (such as spinal cord injuries or neuromuscular diseases), congenital heart disease, hemoglobinopathies (disorders characterized by alterations in the structure of hemoglobin, which often results in anemia), metabolic conditions (such as diabetes), or suppression of the immune system. The incidence of both primary viral pneumonia and secondary bacterial lung infection that results in hospitalization is higher in these at-risk children, and influenza shedding can be prolonged for up to weeks after symptoms resolve. When compared to older patients, children also experience a higher frequency of central nervous complications, which are often associated with very poor outcomes. Thankfully, despite the increased risk of complicated disease, children are usually less likely to die of influenza than adults.

Of note, children are highly contagious with influenza; they may begin shedding the virus days before symptoms even occur and continue to shed the virus for more than 10 days beyond the active phase of illness.

People with Chronic Diseases

People with certain chronic medical conditions, including lung disease (such as asthma), heart problems, metabolic issues (such as diabetes), and extreme obesity are at risk for severe influenza infection. Overall, 31 percent of adults in the United States who are 50–64 years old, and 47 percent of adults in the United States who are 65 years or older, are estimated to be at high risk for influenza complications because of chronic health conditions. In the 2017–2018 flu season, nearly a million people were hospitalized in the United States. Among those, 92 percent had one or more underlying medical conditions that placed them at high risk for influenza-related complications. More specifically, 46 percent had cardiovascular disease, 43 percent had metabolic disorders such as diabetes, 37 percent were obese, and 30 percent had chronic lung disease.

Studies have shown that influenza infection is associated with an increase in heart attacks and stroke. Flu can make diabetes worse because infection makes it harder to control the blood sugar; diabetes also makes the immune system less able to fight against infections. People who suffer from chronic lung disease or asthma can have worsening of their underlying lung process when infected with influenza (people with lung disease or asthma already have swollen and sensitive airways, and influenza can cause this to worsen further). Influenza can trigger asthma attacks, and children and adults with asthma are more likely to develop pneumonia after getting sick with flu than people who do not have asthma. Some studies have shown that the combination of chronic lung disease or asthma with influenza can cause permanent loss of lung function.

A recent survey conducted by the National Foundation for Infectious Diseases (NFID) showed that less than 25 percent of adults in the United States understand that people with heart disease or diabetes are at great risk for influenza-related complications, and awareness was significantly lower among people of color than among white people. Even fewer knew that heart attack, worsening of diabetes, stroke, or other disability can result in potential influenza-related complications.

Elderly Adults

Adults who are 65 years of age or older are at risk for more severe symptoms and even death when infected with influenza, especially if they reside in a nursing home. It is estimated that 70–90 percent of the flu-related deaths, and between 50 and 70 percent of flu-related hospitalizations, during seasonal epidemics each year are in people of this age group.

Factors that contribute to more severe influenza infections in older adults include a diminished cough reflex that is associated with normal aging, decreased compliance of the lungs, deficits in respiratory muscle strength, declining immune system function (especially at the cellular level), decreased antibody response to new antigens, nutritional deficiencies, greater exposures to other sick people due to close living quarters and shared caregivers, and the frequent presence of other medical conditions.

Immunocompromised People

In people whose immune system is compromised by disease or medications, the severity of symptoms may be worse when influenza infection occurs. There is also an increased risk of serious complications such as primary viral pneumonia or secondary bacterial pneumonia, leading to high rates of hospitalization, intensive care unit admission, and death.

People with human immunodeficiency virus (HIV) infection can be at increased risk for heart- and lung-related hospitalizations during influenza season as opposed to other times of the year, and they may have prolonged influenza symptoms when infected. People who have undergone organ or bone marrow transplantation can experience a high likelihood of graft dysfunction and rejection after influenza infection. People with active cancer, or who have survived certain types of cancer such as lymphoma or leukemia, may not necessarily be at more risk of getting the flu, but they are known to be at higher risk of complications from influenza infection.

People who are severely immunocompromised can shed virus for weeks to months after infection. While they might have recovered from their flu symptoms, the viral shedding means that they are able to spread the infection to others, even if they don't feel ill.

Pregnant Women

Both pregnant and postpartum women are known to be at risk for more severe consequences when suffering from the flu due to changes in the immune system, heart, and lungs. Historically, pregnant women have suffered disproportionally during influenza pandemics, and new studies have shown an increasing incidence of hospitalizations in pregnant women during the influenza season for acute heart and lung issues. The risk of hospitalization increases with length of pregnancy and in those with high-risk medical conditions. Influenza infection in pregnant women can also be harmful to the developing baby. Fever that occurs during the flu may be associated with neural tube defects and other bad outcomes for the fetus.

Of note, vaccination is the first and most important step in protecting both mother and baby against the flu. A study in 2018 showed that getting a flu shot reduced a pregnant woman's risk of being hospitalized with flu by an average of 40 percent. Pregnant women who get vaccinated are also helping to protect their baby from flu for the first several months after birth when they are too young to get vaccinated themselves (the maternal antibodies produced in response to the vaccine are passed on to the baby). Despite these impressive statistics and the availability of safe and effective vaccines, the CDC reported in the fall of 2019 that the majority of pregnant women in the United States (about 65 percent of them) had not undergone flu vaccination.

American Indians and Alaska Natives

Flu and pneumonia rank among the top 10 causes of death for American Indians and Alaska Natives, and one study showed that they have almost a twofold increased risk of dying from these infections than other races. American Indians and Alaska Natives are more likely to live in poverty when compared to some other races, and low socioeconomic status could contribute to some of the household and environmental factors that are known to increase risk of respiratory tract infections (such as household crowding, lack of running water, poor indoor air quality with use of wood-burning stoves and suboptimal household ventilation, and rural or remote locations). Other contributors to the increased risk in American Indians and Alaska Natives were tobacco smoking, presence of chronic health conditions, and less access to preventive care (such as vaccines and antiviral medications).

4

Signs and Symptoms

Humans have a defense system that stands ready against invasion by an unwelcome germ like influenza. Even as an inhaled viral particle enters the respiratory tract of a new host, the body is already attempting to limit its chance of harmful infection. Hairs in the nose provide an obstacle that might slow the travel of a viral particle. Saliva itself contains enzymes that try to break down and destroy the virus. Mucus is secreted along the lining of the respiratory tract, trapping anything unwanted and encouraging its path back up the throat to be swallowed or coughed out. The respiratory epithelial cells directly underneath the mucus layer have projections called cilia, which continuously beat in a sweeping motion, trying to remove unwanted germs and debris. The acts of coughing and sneezing attempt to force fluid, mucus, and germs outward. If a virus is able to bypass all of the body's physical defenses, it must attach to and enter the cells lining the respiratory tract before it can begin the production of more viral particles. It is fortunate for influenza, then, that the human respiratory epithelial cells actually have receptors on their surface that recognize and receive the flu virus. It is also to the virus's benefit that enzymes in the host cell are available to assist with entry into the cell and the start of viral replication.

THE HOST IMMUNE RESPONSE

When infected with the influenza virus, the human host has a very clear and identifiable immune response. The degree of illness experienced by the host is dependent on both the strength of their immune system and any past immunity that may have developed in response to previous infection with the flu. The defenses offered by the human immune system are impressive and include both antibody production (known as humoral immunity) and white blood cell responses (known as cellular immunity). Antibodies are proteins that are produced by immune system cells when they come in contact with specific sites (known as antigens) on the surface of a pathogen. Antibodies usually offer long-lasting protection against reinfection with the same germ because, once activated, the immune system cells help in the production of those germ-specific antibodies if and when the infection is recognized again. Thus, hosts that survive an acute viral infection would be expected, for the most part, to be immune to infections by the same virus in the future. Unfortunately, this concept does not hold true with influenza. Because of the virus's tendency to mutate via antigenic drift, humans are unable to produce a perfect antibody response that would prevent infection with all of the various subtypes or strains of the influenza virus from year to year.

In response to initial infection with the flu, antibody formation against the HA and NA glycoproteins, as well as to the membrane and other proteins, occurs in the host; these antibodies are produced both system-wide and locally within the respiratory tract itself. Antibodies produced against HA attempt to neutralize the influenza virus and reduce its ability to enter and infect cells. The antibodies against NA, on the other hand, work to reduce the release of virus from already infected cells; this decreases the severity of host symptoms while also limiting viral shedding. Antibodies produced against membrane and other proteins do not appear to render the virus ineffective, nor do they play a role in protective immunity against future infections. These antibodies do, however, provide a marker that can be measured in the bloodstream of infected patients, which may help in the diagnosis of recent infection. Peak levels of these antibodies can be measured about four to seven weeks after infection, and the levels decline slowly thereafter; however, low levels of antibodies can be detected even years after infection in some people.

In addition to antibody production, the human host has a cellular immune response. T lymphocytes (a type of white blood cell) are activated, and they migrate to the site of infection. One type of T lymphocyte, called CD8, helps kill host cells that have been invaded by the influenza virus; this, in turn, shuts down the viral replication process. Another T lymphocyte type, called CD4, helps with generation of antibodies and activation of immune cells that produce cytokines, which are substances like interferon, tumor necrosis factor, and interleukins. Cytokines have multiple functions, including initiation of an inflammatory cascade. It is this immune response that causes many of the prominent symptoms, such as fever, headache, and muscle aches, which often occur during infection with influenza. Some cytokines force cells to make a variety of proteins in an attempt to halt the virus, including one that prevents viruses from using RNA for replication. Another cytokine acts as a toxin and can be lethal to cells; cell death, in turn, shuts down the production of new viral particles.

Although the immune system response is intended to offer protection to the host, it can also cause great harm once it is activated. At a cellular level, the cytokine toxins that are released in an attempt to destroy infected cells can prove deadly to nearby healthy cells, too. Epithelial cells lining the respiratory tract are killed in great numbers as the immune system attempts to combat the influenza infection, leaving the host with a sore throat. Other immune cells can release a substance that promotes production of more white blood cells that act in the body's defense; unfortunately, activity within the bone marrow during white blood cell production can cause severe pain. While the immune system focuses on eradication of the influenza virus, the body's defenses against bacteria are lessened and secondary bacterial infection of the respiratory tract can occur. Mucus and fluid that are produced along the respiratory tract in response to infection can clog the airways, causing shortness of breath and cough. If the lower respiratory tract becomes involved in the infection, small blood vessels can be destroyed; bleeding or hemorrhaging can result. Debris from dying cells, old blood, and a protective fibrin-like connective tissue produced by lung cells can disrupt the transfer of oxygen between the blood and the lung's air sacs; without enough oxygen, lung tissue begins to die. Finally, the disintegration of lung tissue can result in a clinical condition known as acute respiratory distress syndrome (ARDS), which greatly increases the risk of respiratory failure and death from influenza infection.

As the different strains of influenza have been identified and studied, it has become clear that the cytokine response and the resulting inflammatory cascade of the host may differ depending on the strain of flu causing the infection. For example, it has been suggested that Hong Kong H5N1, identified in 1997, triggered an extremely potent cytokine release, and this may have accounted for the high death rates that occurred in people infected with that strain. The immune response with Hong Kong H5N1 was so impressive that organs even beyond the lungs were affected in fatal cases, including death and destruction of liver cells, evidence of kidney damage, and depletion of white blood cells. A vigorous immune and inflammatory response might have also influenced death rates during the influenza pandemic in 1918, resulting in the loss of a significant number of predominately young and previously healthy adults.

It is clear that the host's immune response, when triggered by infection with the flu, can result in a wide variety of symptoms and, for some people, even death. What, then, are the disease states that are caused by influenza?

UNCOMPLICATED INFLUENZA

In uncomplicated cases of influenza, the symptoms are uncomfortable but rarely fatal. Upon initial infection, the flu virus affects mainly the upper respiratory tract, including the nose, throat, and bronchi (the two divisions of the trachea that lead into the lungs). So, in uncomplicated influenza infection, the most prominent manifestations might include both systemic symptoms triggered by the immune response and localized symptoms within the upper respiratory tract. Onset of symptoms is usually abrupt, and often, people can remember exactly when they started to feel sick. Despite the fact that the influenza virus directly infects the epithelial cells lining the respiratory tract, respiratory symptoms are usually present to a lesser extent than the systemic, or generalized, complaints in uncomplicated influenza. Common systemic symptoms include fever, shaking chills, sweats, headache, muscle aches (especially in the calf muscles and the back), fatigue, poor appetite, bone and joint pains, and even confusion. More localized symptoms related to the upper respiratory tract include tearing and/or burning of the eyes, congestion of the nose, runny nose, sore throat, hoarseness, and dry cough (not associated with production of sputum).

The fever usually lasts about two to three days, although the fever can sometimes persist for four to eight days in some people. The temperature of a person infected with influenza can rise suddenly and can even reach greater than 105 degrees Fahrenheit within 12 hours in some children and adults. The fever is often continuous, but occasionally can be intermittent, especially if medications to aid in fever reduction are used; these types of medications are called antipyretics. In some people, fever that appears to have resolved can come back again on the third or fourth day of symptoms, creating what is called a biphasic fever curve.

Overall, the presence of fever is probably the most important physical finding in identifying an adult with the flu, along with cough. Indeed, the abrupt onset of fever with cough has about a 70 percent chance of representing the flu in an adult if the symptoms occur during a seasonal influenza epidemic. These symptoms are less helpful in identifying influenza in people who have underlying medical conditions, though. For example, one study of clinical predictors of influenza in people who required hospitalization found that fever with cough or sore throat was only correct about 21 percent of the time if they also had asthma. There are other exceptions to the typical influenza symptom pattern as well:

- Older people have higher frequency of confusion.
- Respiratory complaints may not be identifiable in older patients at all during the initial stage of infection, but secondary bacterial pneumonia is more likely to occur.

- Infants or young children and the elderly may not always have fever; however, when feverish, temperatures can reach a higher level in children than in adults.
- A good percentage of infants and young children often have a barking cough and/or diarrhea.
- Swollen and tender lymph nodes at the neck are more common in children.
- Younger patients are more likely to suffer from ear pain, nausea, and vomiting.
- Occasionally, children can have seizure activity when their fever is high; 6–20 percent of children hospitalized with influenza have been reported to have these febrile seizures.
- People with compromised immune systems may have very subtle symptoms as a clue to their illness.

Often the respiratory symptoms in uncomplicated influenza persist for three to four days beyond fever itself. After this phase, some people may take one to two (or more) weeks to entirely recover their original state of health. The last symptoms to go away completely are usually the cough and the sense of fatigue. Adults can spread the flu to others at least a day before they experience any obvious symptoms, and they can shed the virus for up to five to seven days after all of their symptoms have resolved. However, viral shedding can be more extended in children and immunocompromised adults.

The illness caused by influenza A is nearly indistinguishable from the illness caused by influenza B, although typically, it is felt that influenza B infections tend to be milder than those caused by influenza A. Influenza C usually mimics only a common cold and rarely causes the same degree of symptoms as influenza A or B.

COMPLICATED INFLUENZA

Although many of us have experienced the relatively uncomplicated symptoms of flu during seasonal epidemics, the virus can, unfortunately, make some people very sick and may even cause death. The most common complication of influenza is pneumonia, which is an acute inflammation of lung tissue and clogging of the air sacs with white blood cells and debris as a consequence of the infection. Two types of pneumonias can result from infection with the flu: primary viral pneumonia and secondary bacterial pneumonia. Sometimes, a combination of these two types of lung infections can exist at the same time.

Primary Viral Pneumonia

Primary viral pneumonia is an illness that often begins with the symptoms that are common in uncomplicated influenza, such as fever, cough, sore throat, muscle aches, and fatigue. Unfortunately, if the flu virus has managed to involve the lower respiratory tract, these early symptoms can be quickly followed by a rapid progression to shortness of breath, increased work of breathing, and an inability to transport oxygen as needed to vital tissues. The lack of oxygen results in a bluish color and can best be seen at the lips, fingers, and toes; this condition is known as cyanosis. These manifestations suggest the complication of primary viral pneumonia.

It is somewhat difficult to identify who may progress from uncomplicated influenza to primary viral pneumonia. It is known that it happens more often in people with underlying heart (specifically, stenosis of the mitral valve) or lung diseases (such as asthma); it also occurs more in pregnant women. However, it is now thought that many of the deaths in young, healthy adults that occurred during the influenza pandemics in 1918 and 1957 were due to primary viral pneumonia, perhaps because of specific viral factors that influenced the immune response and resulting inflammatory cascade.

Clinically, people with suspected or confirmed influenza infection who have decreased oxygen saturation measurements (indicating that tissues are not being adequately oxygenated), breathing rates greater than 25 times per minute, diarrhea, or low blood pressure readings, may be more likely to be progressing toward primary viral pneumonia. Sputum output during coughing that shows evidence of blood is also a worrisome symptom. Upon evaluation in a medical setting, people found to have abnormal laboratories, such as elevated lactate dehydrogenase, creatine phosphokinase, creatinine, and c-reactive protein, are considered to have more severe disease. Chest x-rays often show abnormalities of the lower respiratory tract, but results can be difficult to distinguish from other causes such as fluid in the lungs and/or pleural space.

The risk of death in people who progress from uncomplicated influenza to primary viral pneumonia is high, in part because of the potential for ARDS. If this occurs, there is usually worsening of shortness of breath and severe oxygenation issues with a cough resulting in a thin, bloody sputum that shows few cells. Respiratory failure requiring intubation for mechanical ventilation usually results, often after only one day of hospitalization. When autopsies are performed on people who have died from primary viral pneumonia, inflammation along the respiratory tract at the trachea, the bronchial tree, and into the alveolar ducts can be seen, and evidence of bleeding can be found. At the level of the air sacs of the lungs, however, few inflammatory cells exist. Unfortunately, because the pneumonia is due to the influenza virus itself, antibiotics are not effective (antibiotics have killing activity against bacteria, but not against viruses). Management of people who have primary viral pneumonia involves a combination of antiviral treatment targeting the influenza virus and supportive care, which can include ventilatory support, adequate fluid balance, and nutritional aid. Some people with severe cases of primary viral pneumonia who don't respond to usual measures may require a special type of respiratory support called venovenous extracorporeal membrane oxygenation (known as ECMO) or even prone positioning in bed.

Secondary Bacterial Pneumonia

The second type of pneumonia that can complicate an infection with influenza is not caused by the virus itself, but rather by another germ: bacteria that manages to infect the lower respiratory tract at the same time (or shortly thereafter) the upper and/or lower tract is infected by the flu. While the host's immune system is occupied with fighting the influenza virus, it can leave the person less protected against another lung infection. The flu virus inhibits adequate action of the disease-fighting white blood cells in the lungs themselves, and there is also evidence that the virus helps some bacteria's ability to attach to lung tissue and cause infection. So, if the host (already infected with influenza) is exposed to bacteria that prefers to invade and infect respiratory cells, it may not be able to avoid another new infection. The most common bacterial coinfection associated with influenza is *Streptococcus pneumoniae*; however, *Staphylococcus aureus* and *Streptococcus pyogenes* (the same germ that causes strep throat) have often been found as culprits causing secondary bacterial pneumonia as well.

The patients who tend to suffer from secondary bacterial pneumonia are often at the extremes of age and may be ill with other diseases such as heart, lung, or metabolic problems. While bacterial coinfection with influenza can already be present when people seek medical attention, it is not uncommon for it to develop later. People may have an identifiable illness attributable to influenza first and show a brief period of recovery (this period is often two to three days in length, but it can be up to two weeks). Then, they will have recurrent symptoms that can include fever, cough, production of sputum that resembles pus, and difficulty breathing due to the bacterial invasion.

Unfortunately, there are few tools or diagnostic measures that can reliably tell the difference between people who have solely a viral infection versus infection with both influenza and bacteria. People with development of secondary bacterial pneumonia usually look quite ill. On medical evaluation, they might have signs of infection deep into the lungs that can be heard through a stethoscope. Their sputum, when evaluated in the laboratory, can show a predominance of white blood cells and bacteria, often with one bacterial strain in the majority as the infecting pathogen. As with primary viral pneumonia, they may have laboratory abnormalities that reflect severe infection (elevated lactic acid, increased white blood cell count, increased or decreased platelet count, elevated c-reactive protein and procalcitonin, and increased creatinine). Chest x-ray and/or computed tomography scan of the chest show lung abnormalities that are consistent with lower respiratory tract infection.

People suffering from secondary bacterial pneumonia can also progress to severe respiratory disease, including ARDS with a need for mechanical ventilatory support. An overwhelming bacterial infection can cause complications beyond the lungs with involvement of the blood stream and strain on other organ systems. However, because bacteria can be targeted and treated with antibiotic therapy, people with secondary bacterial pneumonia often get better with supportive care and appropriate antimicrobial medications.

It has been proposed that, in addition to the prevalence of primary viral pneumonia, the severity of the second wave of the 1918 influenza pandemic (and the tendency for the virus to kill young, healthy adults) was attributable to the possible synergy between the virus itself and a complicating bacterium. In the more recent influenza pandemic of 2009, bacterial coinfection may have been more prevalent than initially thought. A recent analysis of lung specimens from 77 people who died during the 2009 pandemic found that 29 percent showed evidence of a concurrent bacterial pneumonia; the most common bacterial pathogens were *Streptococcal pneumoniae*, *Staphylococcus aureus*, and *Streptococcus pyogenes*.

EXTRAPULMONARY MANIFESTATIONS

Though less frequent than the complication of pneumonia, manifestations of influenza have been described in organs beyond the lungs. For example, descriptions of people suffering from the flu during the 1918 pandemic were severe and all encompassing. People were noted to have both mental and physical neurological consequences like delirium with mental depression, hysteria, melancholy, suicidal thoughts, and paralysis. Some had extreme ear pain with perforation of the ear drum. Hemorrhaging of blood from the nose, mouth, ears, eyes, lungs, bowel, and vagina was described. On examination, doctors found subcutaneous emphysema, or pockets of air that accumulated just beneath the skin that was heard to "crackle" when pressed. Some people lost the ability to move their eyes or even smell. Others suffered from chest pain and were likely to have had heart attacks. Extrapulmonary manifestations will be discussed in more detail in chapter 6.

5

Diagnosis, Management, and Treatment

All of the symptoms that come with infection due to influenza can make a person feel miserable, and in some cases, the illness can progress to a more complicated disease or even death. It is not unexpected, then, for many people to seek medical attention with a health care provider, hoping for both clarification of their diagnosis and discussion about possible treatment options.

MEDICAL PROVIDER VISIT

With knowledge gleaned from years of study and clinical training, as well as general wisdom that comes with both age and experience, a good medical provider should be able to identify the signs and symptoms suggestive of influenza. The initial approach to evaluating a person who might be sick with the flu includes taking a health history and conducting a physical examination. The information obtained during the history and physical then guide the provider in making decisions about laboratory testing or radiology studies that might help confirm the diagnosis. Once a diagnosis is made, management strategies and treatment alternatives can be considered.

Health History

The health history is essentially the story, told by the person who is ill (or by knowledgeable friends, family, and/or caregivers), outlining current symptoms and past medical problems. The history varies a great degree in terms of details and is, of course, dependent upon the age of the patient and their ability to communicate with others. The health history taken from a person sick with the flu could consist of several core components, including the following:

- Chief complaint: A short description of the primary reason for seeking medical attention. For example, a patient sick with influenza might tell their provider, "I have a fever, sore throat, and my head and back hurt a lot."
- History of present illness: A more detailed, chronological account of the illness, with particular attention paid to the location, quality, severity, and timing of the symptoms. People sick with the flu should share when they first began to feel ill (exact timing of the start of symptoms is very important because it influences whether or not certain antiviral treatments might be offered), what various symptoms they have experienced, and how the symptoms progressed over time.
- Past medical history: A list of prior health problems, including illnesses, hospitalizations, or accidents and injuries. Because people with certain conditions and diseases can be at increased risk of complications from influenza, providers need to be aware of this background history.
- Past surgical history: A list of previous procedures, interventions, or operations. Though this might seem to be unrelated to the flu, certain surgeries can influence the risk of complications with influenza (e.g., removal of a portion of lung or need for a chronic breathing tube called a tracheostomy) or a patient's immune response to infection (such as previous removal of the spleen).
- Allergies: A list of the person's medication allergies or reactions to vaccination, especially with regard to antibiotics, antiviral medications, and the influenza vaccine. It is also relevant to ask about food allergies, as egg allergies often warrant clarification when considering recommendations for influenza vaccination.
- Medications: A list of any home remedies and both nonprescription and prescription drugs that the person is currently taking. This list helps clarify whether the person might be immunocompromised because of certain drugs or if there could be interactions between medications if antimicrobial treatment is prescribed.

- Family history: Age and health status (or cause of death) of close family members, including any current sick contacts that might also be suffering from the flu.
- Social history: Documentation of behavioral and psychosocial information, such as employment, marriage status, home situation, tobacco use, alcohol use, or illicit drug use. Some of these issues are known to contribute to greater risk of complications in people infected with influenza.
- Review of systems: An assessment of the systems of the body in an attempt to identify diagnostic clues that might not have been covered in the history of present illness. This quick review helps medical providers focus on signs and symptoms that are clues to influenza infection that might not have been readily shared by the patient as they told their story.

During their training, medical providers are actually taught specific interviewing techniques that can help them gather accurate information from people who are seeking their help, especially since people who are sick don't always feel like talking and are more likely to share their story if the provider acts in an empathetic and efficient manner. One practice used by medical providers is to begin the conversation with general, open-ended questions. This allows the person on the exam table to offer a response in whatever way they prefer and gives the person a chance to talk freely. Providers are aware that they should withhold interruptions during the history of present illness. Studies have confirmed that medical providers can be quick to interrupt their patients. (One medical study has shown that physicians, on average, listen to their patients' concerns for about 18 seconds before interrupting; however, on average, a patient will take two and a half minutes to tell their story completely if they aren't interrupted.) It is stressed during medical training that a more accurate health history is the key to a more accurate diagnosis and that the health history is dependent on how well a person can complete their story in their own words. Once a person has given their history, the provider might then ask some clarifying questions. These further questions offer the best chance at a helpful response if they aren't intended to only elicit "yes" or "no." Questions that require a graded answer (for example, "How far can you walk before you get short of breath?") are likely to be more helpful than asking "Do you get short of breath when you walk?" It is also preferable for the medical provider to ask one question at a time, rather than rattling off a list of symptoms all at once. Finally, a good provider will always end the conversation with "Is there anything else about your illness that you think I need to know?" as a prompt for any forgotten details.

There are actually a number of things that you, as a patient, can do when visiting your medical provider to practice good patient etiquette, which can, in turn, improve the dialogue between you and your provider during the evaluation and help lead to more accurate diagnosis and treatment outcomes. Establishing a good rapport and mutual trust with your medical provider can also result in a more fulfilling and beneficial interaction for both you and them. Some good patient etiquette techniques to consider include the following:

- Before the appointment, spend some time reviewing the symptoms you'd like to share with your provider, especially in terms of timing and severity.
- Limit the visit to the current illness, and if there are more issues beyond the flu that you'd like to be addressed, schedule another visit.
- Give the history of present illness in a concise, clear manner and answer questions truthfully.
- Display a positive attitude and consider asking the provider, "What can I do to make myself feel better?"
- Avoid comments that might signal a sense of distrust and try not to criticize other medical providers or personnel.
- Don't attempt to influence your provider's diagnosis or treatment with the use of anecdotal experiences about other patients or doctors. Also, don't withhold information about important sick contacts.
- Think about what your provider would be expected to do with any outside information brought to the visit from the library, television, or internet; trust that your provider knows where to find the most updated and relevant medical information about influenza and other illnesses.
- Try not to expect the impossible and keep expectations realistic. Remember that antibiotics don't work against viral infections and that your provider is right not to prescribe them if your diagnosis is the flu.
- Don't ask your provider to do something unethical or illegal.

Physical Examination

The symptoms that accompany an infection like influenza have associated physical clues that can be found on examination of the body. A skillful medical provider will be thorough yet efficient, systematic but not rigid, and gentle but competent when completing an exam. The degree of examination depends upon the story heard during the health history; a targeted examination of the respiratory system might be enough to diagnose a case of uncomplicated influenza, but a more thorough evaluation would be indicated for a person who shared a history that was worrisome for a more complicated infection.

The physical examination often begins with a review of the vital signs, including temperature, heart rate, respiratory rate, blood pressure, and weight. Concern for a respiratory infection such as influenza might also prompt measurement of the oxygen level in the blood. With influenza, the temperature is often elevated, indicating a fever. The heart rate and respiratory rate might also be increased, because of both the fever and the body's immune response to infection. Blood pressure readings can be either high or low in the setting of active infection, though low readings are often more worrisome. People sometimes have weight loss during a bout of the flu, particularly if they have had poor appetite along with nausea and vomiting or diarrhea.

The remaining components of the physical examination (and some of the findings that might result from influenza infection) are as follows:

- General survey: Overall appearance and state of mind; people with influenza can look quite ill (especially in the setting of active fever), may appear tired, or even be somewhat confused.
- Skin: Sweat and flushing of the skin, along with feelings of warmth, can accompany fever, while cyanosis (a cold, bluish tinge caused by poor oxygen exchange) can sometimes be seen in severe infection, especially at the lips, fingers, and/or toes.
- Head/eyes/ears/nose/throat (HEENT): The eyes can be red and watery, the nose can sound congested or show obvious drainage of mucus, the tissues inside the nose can look swollen, and the throat can be red and irritated. The voice may even be hoarse.
- Neck: Enlarged lymph nodes can be felt along the front and back of the neck and can be tender to the touch, especially in children.
- Lungs: A "crackling" sound can sometimes be heard when listening to the lungs through a stethoscope due to air attempting to travel through congestion. Some people experience chest pain when breathing deeply; this is known as pleurisy. A dullness heard when tapping the back over the region of the lungs can sometimes indicate a lower respiratory tract complication such as secondary bacterial pneumonia or associated pleural fluid infection.
- Heart: The heart rate is often faster than normal in people sick with the flu, and occasionally, an abnormal rhythm can be heard through the stethoscope as a warning of a more worrisome complication. If the heart is beating strongly and quickly (especially during fever), some

medical providers may be able to hear a flow murmur or an atypical sound of blood moving through the heart valve(s).

- Stomach: The abdominal muscles can be tender to palpation if people have had trouble with nausea and dry heaves or vomiting, but it would be unusual to find enlargement of the liver or spleen in people with the flu.
- Musculoskeletal: Both muscle aches (known as myalgias) and joint pain (known as arthralgias) can be exhibited during the medical provider's touch or movement of the spine, arms, or legs.
- Neurologic: The findings of confusion, extreme fatigue, dulled sensibility, or varying degrees of paralysis can be identified as complications of influenza.

Just as there are recommendations for patient etiquette with the health history, there are tips that can help you during a physical examination with your medical provider as well. Consider these factors regarding the exam:

- It is not uncommon or abnormal to feel uncomfortable when you have to disrobe, uncover various parts of your body, or be touched in places that hurt or cause embarrassment during a physical examination.
- It is not unusual for your medical provider to wear gloves during the entire examination. The gloves are not meant to cause alarm or to make you feel alienated or isolated; rather, they are simply a part of standard medical precautions.
- Try not to voice a list of important concerns during the examination itself. The medical provider needs to concentrate as they use the stethoscope to listen to your heart and lungs.
- If you'd like to have your medical provider explain each part of the examination while it is being performed, ask in advance rather than while the exam is being conducted.
- Do not be surprised if your medical provider asks additional questions during certain parts of the examination. These questions do not necessarily imply that they have found something of concern, but instead might indicate that they are supplementing the information they gathered during the earlier health history.
- You should feel comfortable asking questions about findings when your medical provider has finished the physical examination.

Another helpful piece of information for medical providers as they attempt to make the diagnosis of influenza is the knowledge of the virus's activity in the region at the time of the visit. When the presence of seasonal influenza has been confirmed in a community, most patients who present with a flu-like illness to their medical provider will truly have the flu. The accuracy of the clinical diagnosis alone, without any complementary laboratory or radiology testing, in the midst of an influenza outbreak can reach 80–90 percent.

Studies have attempted to identify parameters of the health history and physical examination that might allow for a more accurate diagnosis of influenza. One study showed that three key clinical variables (fever, shaking chills, and sweats) that began less than three days before the person sought medical attention were likely to correlate with true influenza infection. Arguing against influenza as the correct diagnosis were a lack of systemic symptoms such as fever, no report of cough, the ability to cope with activities of daily living, and not being confined to bed. Another recent study specifically evaluated people over 65 years of age or those who had underlying heart and/or lung disease and were admitted to the hospital with a respiratory illness. Twenty percent of these people had influenza, and the best predictor was the combination of cough, fever, and symptoms for seven days or less.

Uncomplicated influenza usually does not require any imaging to aid in the diagnosis. A smart and attentive medical provider will likely be able to diagnose influenza after gathering the health history and doing a focused physical examination. Occasionally, however, use of an imaging study may help either confirm or rule out the diagnosis of complicated influenza. An x-ray of the chest can show abnormalities suggestive of either primary viral pneumonia or secondary bacterial pneumonia. Computed tomography of the chest, which allows a three-dimensional picture, can reveal further complications of influenza in the lung and pleural space. A tracing of the heart rhythm, known as an electrocardiogram (EKG), might be ordered if a savvy medical provider heard an abnormal heart rhythm on examination. Appreciating a heart murmur during the physical examination could also prompt an order for an echocardiogram, which is an ultrasound that provides a visual recording of the heart and its movements. Rarely, more invasive testing may be considered, such as a spinal tap to look for neurological consequences of influenza.

LABORATORY DIAGNOSIS

Though the health history and physical examination might be all that is needed to diagnose influenza in some people, there is sometimes value in confirming the diagnosis with laboratory testing. It has been found that laboratory confirmation of influenza can lead to more appropriate treatment decisions and can help in avoidance of inappropriate management (such as giving antibiotics for a viral infection since antibiotics only have activity against bacteria). The laboratory diagnosis of influenza is also important in helping to prevent, contain, and monitor the illness during seasonal outbreaks and epidemics. With concerns about a future influenza pandemic, the ability to use the laboratory to isolate and subtype the virus allows for better epidemiological surveillance and aids in the production of appropriate vaccines.

Historically, laboratory testing for the flu was not considered to be of much value to medical providers because there was a lengthy wait for test results, the tests weren't perfect (they weren't always positive, even when people really had the flu), and there were few treatment options (such as antiviral medications) to offer even if the diagnosis was confirmed. Now, however, the development of more rapid and accurate tests for influenza gives medical providers a way to almost instantly confirm the diagnosis of flu. This has resulted in more timely initiation of antiviral therapies, avoidance of antibiotics when they aren't helpful, implementation of infection control measures that help stop the spread of flu, decreased need and length of hospitalization, reduction in other unnecessary laboratory and radiology testing, and decreased overall health care costs. Experts recommend that testing for influenza should be performed when the results are anticipated to influence clinical management (e.g., help in decisions to start antiviral or antibiotic treatment, proceed with other testing, or recommend infection control measures) or to influence public health response (such as outbreak identification and intervention). A medical provider's decision to treat is thus based on their level of suspicion for the flu, known local activity with the virus, and the availability of influenza test results. The Infectious Disease Society of America (IDSA) has published clinical guidelines for influenza, including a helpful algorithm that aids medical providers in determining the need for laboratory testing of the flu; the algorithm can be found at https://academic.oup.com/view-large/figure/131800601/ciy86601.jpg.

Viral Culture

Although the flow of mucus from the nose or the production of phlegm from a cough might be uncomfortable for people who are sick with the flu, these body fluids can actually be tested for the presence of the influenza virus. A swab from the nose or throat, washings taken from nasal passages, or a collection of sputum produced by cough can be put into a special vial of viral transport medium and sent to the laboratory where it is processed by viral culture (a means of growing the virus for identification). This is actually the only test that can confirm that viable influenza virus is present in a specimen. Of all the specimen types, the throat swab is the least likely to result in a positive culture; the other specimens have a tendency for higher yield. More than 90 percent of positive cultures can be detected within three days of inoculation, and the remainder of cultures turn positive in five to seven days. Obviously, the time required for a viral culture to turn positive is the downside to such testing: by the time the diagnosis of influenza is made with a viral culture, a patient could be beyond the window of opportunity for antiviral treatment. False-negative results (a negative culture result despite the presence of influenza infection) can occur because of several reasons, including low quantities of the viral particle in some collected respiratory samples, inappropriate collection/handling/transporting of the samples, the presence of viral inhibitors, or the emergence of new viral subtypes for which the culture medium was not designed. False-positive findings (a positive culture despite lack of infection with influenza) can also occur, and this can be due to laboratory error or suboptimal design of the test in question.

Since growing a virus in special medium takes too long to be helpful when people are seeking attention for flu symptoms with their medical provider, viral culture is more often used to provide specific information about circulating strains and subtypes of seasonal influenza A and influenza B viruses. This is particularly important from a public health perspective since knowledge of circulating strains helps in decisions about influenza vaccine selection. Viral cultures can also be used to confirm negative test results for influenza from other methods (this is especially helpful during institutional outbreaks) or to provide influenza virus isolates for further characterization.

Rapid Antigen Tests

Luckily, over time, more rapid testing techniques for influenza became available; the first of these tests were known as rapid antigen tests. These tests are based on an immunological concept: the detection of viral antigen in respiratory secretions by interaction with a specific antibody. In the easy-to-use, self-contained rapid antigen test, a sample of respiratory secretions is treated with an agent to break apart mucus and then tested, on a filter paper, in an optical device or with a dipstick, for a color change reaction that signifies the binding of an antibody to an influenza antigen. In a somewhat similar manner, another type of rapid antigen test detects the presence of viral NA activity in a respiratory sample by using a pigmented substrate.

The rapid antigen tests are designed to detect both influenza A and influenza B strains, are fairly simple to perform in the lab, and can provide a result within 15 minutes. If the respiratory specimen was obtained with accuracy and care, the tests can report a true positive result about 40–80 percent of the time. The test is most accurate in young children and older people early in their illness (probably because they shed much larger quantities of virus in their respiratory secretions). These tests are most likely to be successful if performed on collections from the nose and/or throat by aspiration rather than swabs or gargles. It has been shown that the ability to use these rapid tests where medical providers are seeing their patients (for instance, in the medical office or urgent care center) can reduce costs by limiting the use of inappropriate treatments, decreasing orders for blood cultures, and allowing avoidance of unnecessary chest x-rays. Given the range in actually providing true positive results, though, the primary issue with the rapid antigen tests is the false-negative probability. False-negative results are more likely to occur if the respiratory specimen was collected more than four days after the start of symptoms. Because of this, it is not recommended that these tests be used on people with progressive illness or in people who have been hospitalized.

Nucleic Acid Testing

Since the rapid antigen tests for influenza can have a decent chance of being false-negative, newer methods known as nucleic acid testing have been developed. These rapid molecular assays, also known as multiplex polymerase chain reaction (PCR) or RT-PCR tests, are based on amplification of the influenza virus RNA by reverse-transcription PCR or nucleic acid sequence-based amplification. They can be used to identify influenza A or influenza B strains, and depending on the type of assay used, results can be available in as little as 15 minutes (though some other assays may take up to eight hours). These are sensitive tests and can even allow the diagnosis of influenza in tissue or other specimens in which the virus has lost its viability. These tests are more labor intensive, are technically demanding, require special equipment, and are potentially more expensive to perform; however, they have replaced the viral culture as the reference standard and are now recommended as a confirmation test when rapid antigen testing is negative in people suspected of having influenza infection. In addition, it is recommended that these assays always be used in hospitalized patients. Another benefit to nucleic acid testing is that they can more readily identify influenza viruses in immunosuppressed transplant patients and in people with chronic lung disease; these patient groups have been difficult to test in the past because of low levels of the virus along the respiratory tract despite obvious illness.

Immunofluorescence Microscopy

Also known as a direct fluorescent antibody test or an immunofluorescent antibody test, this method of testing involves staining of respiratory epithelial cells with specific antibodies, which are linked to a fluorescent dye. These tests can look for both influenza A and influenza B strains, and they can be completed in about one to four hours. Though the immunofluorescence technique is a bit less likely to result in false-negative tests than the rapid antigen tests, the performance depends heavily on laboratory expertise and the quality of the specimen collected. The respiratory specimen must have an adequate number of infected cells for accuracy; in addition, this test requires a special florescent microscope and an experienced laboratory technician to ensure proper implementation and interpretation.

Serological Testing

Once the illness caused by influenza is over, the chance of making a diagnosis by clinical evaluation or rapid testing is low. Luckily, there is a way to find evidence of influenza infection in the blood by measuring antibody levels; this is known as serological testing. The first specimen of blood is drawn within two weeks of the illness (known as the acute phase), followed by a second sample of blood drawn several weeks later (called the convalescent phase). By obtaining these paired blood samples, a rise in antibody levels can be detected over time, which would suggest that infection has occurred. A single specimen of blood sent for antibody testing is not particularly helpful because most people have been exposed to influenza at some point during their lifetime; this leaves a baseline level of antibody that can be detected at any random point in time. Instead, a fourfold or more rise in the influenza antibody levels between the acute phase and the convalescent phase of illness is diagnostic of infection. In addition, serologic testing can be used to measure the response to influenza vaccination because there should be a rise in antibody levels after the vaccine has been administered.

Additional Labs

Along with the testing that allows for the diagnosis of influenza infection in and of itself, there are other laboratory evaluations that might provide clues to infection, particularly if the clinical course is complicated. Blood tests can be performed to look for an elevated white blood cell reaction, which is often an indicator of infection (although in some people, the white blood cell count can actually drop during a viral infection). Another type of blood cell, known as platelets, can be either elevated or abnormally low in the setting of infection. Certain chemistries measured in the blood can be elevated during influenza infection, including lactate dehydrogenase, creatine phosphokinase, creatinine, c-reactive protein, and lactic acid. Blood cultures can be drawn in an attempt to grow bacteria or fungus; if positive, these cultures could provide evidence of an alternative diagnosis or a secondary infection. Analysis of oxygen exchange in the blood can verify concerns for severe pulmonary involvement, especially if cyanosis was seen on examination. Spinal fluid analysis can reveal reaction to the virus in the central nervous system. Liver enzyme testing can be a clue to the occurrence of Reye's syndrome (a rare but serious syndrome that causes swelling in the liver and brain).

MANAGEMENT AND TREATMENT

Historically, there was little to offer to people who became infected with the flu. Both medical providers and people who were suffering from symptoms tried "scientific" remedies and preventives that were touted to be beneficial. Healers proposed that people should undergo vigorous antiseptic cleansing rituals. Community fountains were sterilized with blowtorches, and public telephones were wiped with alcohol. Teeth were pulled and tonsils were removed in the hope that infection could be surgically removed. Steam vapor mixed with eucalyptus or camphor was inhaled. Schools, churches, and theaters were closed; quarantines were attempted. Emergency hospitals were created to help house sick patients. Luckily, identification of the influenza virus, along with a greater understanding of its viral structure, ultimately allowed researchers to develop more effective treatments and preventative medications. As of yet, however, a true cure for influenza does not exist.

Supportive Care

For many people with uncomplicated influenza, all that is needed to recover from the illness is short-term bed rest, good hydration, and time; the person's immune system does all the rest. For some, however, there are other supportive treatments can be used to help in alleviation of specific symptoms:

- Ingestion of medications can offer relief from pain due to headache or muscle discomfort (analgesics) or fever (antipyretics). Note, however, that aspirin must be avoided in people who are 18 years of age or younger due to the association with Reye's syndrome.

- Sprays or drops can be used to treat congestion and obstruction of the passages of the nose. Decongestant sprays should only be used for three consecutive days, or a phenomenon known as rebound congestion might occur (expansion of the tiny blood vessels in the nose, leading to worsening feelings of congestion, which can then prompt a cycle of more and more use of the spray). If sneezing is a problem, sometimes an antihistamine can help.
- Gargling with a mixture of water and salt two to three times a day can sometimes offer temporary relief of a sore throat or hoarse voice, and there are throat sprays that can transiently minimize pain at the back of the throat.
- Suppressants to ease or alleviate cough can be used. Liquid suppressants with dextromethorphan or codeine often work well if used as directed (however, medications that include codeine require a prescription).
- Attention to nutrition with light meals that are easy to digest, hot tea, a glass of orange juice daily, and avoidance of high-fat foods is recommended. Some people find that gastrointestinal symptoms can be eased with carbonated beverages such as ginger ale.
- Fluid repletion with intravenous access may be necessary if severe dehydration occurs. Replacement of electrolytes like sodium and potassium can occasionally be needed, especially if food and water intake is limited because of vomiting or diarrhea.
- Administration of oxygen and, in severe cases, consideration of intubation for use of mechanical ventilation to assist with breathing might be needed.

In addition to these supportive measures, another key component of care that shouldn't be ignored is infection control. Simple acts such as proper hand hygiene, cough etiquette (e.g., covering the mouth while coughing with the elbow and upper arm instead of the hands), and avoidance of others who are sick to limit exposure can have a significant impact on decreasing the spread of the flu and reducing the risk of severe disease in people who are at higher risk when sick.

Medications

There are a number of antiviral medications that are now available for use in people who have infection with influenza. Most people with an intact immune system who become infected with the flu readily trigger their host defenses and limit the amount of viral replication on their own.

So, the opportunity to influence any further viral replication with medicines is somewhat limited; effective use of antiviral medications thus requires early initiation. The greatest effect of antiviral medications has been demonstrated when they are started within the first 24 hours of symptoms.

Given the limitations of the antiviral medications, the goal of treatment is not actually to effect a cure. A main reason to consider treatment with an antiviral medication is to lessen the severity and/or length of the flu symptoms and to attempt avoidance of additional complications in high-risk people. Another reason to be aggressive with antiviral treatment is to decrease the spread of the virus; studies have shown that use of antiviral medications may end viral shedding sooner. It is also hoped that aggressive treatment will abort the emergence of a new influenza A subtype (which is the concern for the possibility of a future pandemic).

As previously mentioned, the IDSA published an updated clinical practice guideline for seasonal influenza in 2018. These guidelines suggest use of antiviral treatment as early as possible for confirmed or suspected influenza, regardless of vaccine history, in people who

- are hospitalized;
- have severe or progressive illness;
- are at high risk of complications;
- are aged < 2 years or >= 65 years; and
- are pregnant or within two weeks postpartum.

Treatment is also recommended for consideration in other people based on the clinical judgment of their medical providers. In particular, treatment might be appropriate for those who are not at high risk for complications but who have any of the following criteria:

- Seen in the outpatient setting with illness onset <= two days before presentation
- Symptomatic outpatients with household contacts who are at high risk of developing complications from influenza (particularly those who are immunocompromised)
- Health care providers who are symptomatic and have contacts who are high risk for development of complications from influenza.

Unfortunately, despite these recommendations for use of antiviral medications, a study of 6004 outpatients in the U.S. Flu Vaccine Effectiveness Network during the 2013–2014 season has suggested that early initiation of antiviral therapy is not happening as often as it is indicated. The study showed that only 15 percent of high-risk patients who presented early

Table 5.1 Antiviral Medications Recommended for Treatment of Influenza

Antiviral Name	Route of Administration	Age Recommendation	Dosing/Frequency
M2 Inhibitors	No longer recommended		
Neuraminidase Inhibitors			
Oseltamivir	Oral	2 weeks and older	75 mg twice a day for five days; age- and weight-based dosing for ages 2 weeks to 12 years
Zanamivir	Inhaled	7 years and older	10 mg (two 5 mg inhalations) twice a day for five days
Peramivir	Intravenous	2 years and older	600 mg once
Endonuclease Inhibitors			
Baloxavir marboxil	Oral	12 years and older	Weight 40 to <80 kg: 40 mg once; >= 80 kg: 80 mg once

were prescribed an antiviral drug; this increased to 43 percent in those who had laboratory confirmation of their infection. Only 30 percent of patients not at high risk with early presentation and confirmed influenza were treated.

There are now three classes of antiviral medications that work against influenza: M2 inhibitors, neuraminidase inhibitors, and endonuclease inhibitors (see Table 5.1); there are six antiviral drugs within these classes that have been approved for treating influenza in the United States.

M2 Inhibitors

As was discussed in chapter 1, the influenza virus contains several M proteins. M1 is involved in the structural matrix of the viral particle, while the M2 protein is an ion channel pump known to help maintain the acidic conditions that allow the viral genetic blueprint to move into the nucleus of a host cell, where viral replication then occurs. The drugs known as M2 inhibitors exert their effect on the influenza virus by inhibiting the ion channel pump. Without use of this pump, the virus cannot shed its outer coat and thus cannot enter into the host cell's nucleus. If the influenza virus doesn't reach the nucleus, it cannot use the host cell's machinery to make more viruses. Interestingly, even though influenza B and C viruses appear to have similar protein pumps, they are just different enough that M2 inhibitors don't appear to work on any strains except those of influenza A.

Within the class of M2 inhibitors, there are two drugs that are currently available: amantadine and rimantadine. Both drugs are available as oral medications that can be ingested. Like the similarities in their names, these medications are related to each other in terms of structure; however, there are still a few notable differences between amantadine and rimantadine. Amantadine, unlike rimantadine, does not undergo metabolic change during ingestion by the human body, and it is eventually excreted unchanged in the urine. Rimantadine undergoes extensive metabolism after it is ingested, and less than 15 percent of the drug is excreted unchanged in the urine. This distinction is important when considering dosing in people who have kidney problems or in the elderly, who can have worsening kidney function with age. Side effects can occur with both amantadine and rimantadine; some of the most common symptoms from these medications are nausea, dizziness, and insomnia. Rimantadine tends to cause less side effects to the central nervous system than amantadine, and there are no known drug interactions with the use of rimantadine.

Amantadine was studied extensively during the pandemic of 1968 with the viral strain H3N2. When taken by people within the first two days of illness, amantadine reduced the duration of fever by about 24 hours. People treated with amantadine also reported more rapid improvement in cough, sore throat, and nasal congestion. In the late 1970s, additional trials of amantadine therapy were performed with the H1N1 strain; similar results were noted then, too. Adults who had taken amantadine showed a more rapid decrease in fever and improved symptoms at 48 hours when compared to people who were given a placebo (a preparation designed to look like medicine, but that has no effect on the body). People treated with amantadine were also less likely to shed virus. Studies with rimantadine showed similar success. People treated with rimantadine during infection with H1N1 and H3N2 viral strains had improved symptoms, decreased fever, and reduced viral shedding when compared with people who took a placebo. Rimantadine has also been studied in children and has been shown to reduce the level of viral shedding early in infection; however, it is not licensed for use in children in the United States.

Unfortunately, despite the benefits that the M2 inhibitors can offer to people infected with influenza A, drug resistance has been a major factor in limiting their use. Up until 2003, reported resistance of the influenza virus to either amantadine or rimantadine was rare, but it has increased remarkably since that time. Resistant viruses are not usually seen in people who haven't been previously exposed to the medications, but they emerge fairly frequently in people who have been treated, especially children.

Resistance is usually the result of mutations in the M2 protein itself, and once the necessary mutations are present, resistance to both drugs is unfortunately guaranteed. Currently, both amantadine and rimantadine are no longer recommended as medications to use for the treatment of influenza A in the United States because of the high level of amantadine resistance among circulating viral strains in recent years.

Neuraminidase Inhibitors

Another class of antiviral medications that work against the flu are the neuraminidase inhibitors. NA is necessary for full penetration of the influenza virus into a host cell and for separation of a newly created viral particle from that cell. With inhibition of the NA molecule by this class of medications, newly created viruses can't detach from their host cell, infect other cells, or make further viral particles to help perpetuate infection. There are three medications currently available in the neuraminidase inhibitor category in the United States: oseltamivir, zanamivir, and peramivir.

Oseltamivir is approved for treatment of people two weeks of age and older, and it comes in both capsules and a powder that can be added to water. It is rapidly absorbed from the gastrointestinal tract as a prodrug and then converted in the liver to an active drug; the active drug is then excreted unchanged via the urine. The dosing has to be adjusted in people with kidney diseases. Zanamivir is supplied as a dry powder for inhalation and cannot be swallowed in pill or solution form. It is excreted unchanged in the urine, with full excretion of a single dose completed in a day. It is recommended for people seven years and older. It has to be administered with fast-acting inhalers nearby for people with underlying lung diseases like asthma because it can worsen breathing, but zanamivir doesn't require dosage adjustment for people with kidney trouble. Peramivir is only available as an infusion that is delivered through the veins, and it is approved for people two years of age and older. If a person with influenza is too sick to swallow or cannot inhale a powder, then peramivir is an alternative way to deliver an antiviral medication. Each of the medications in this class has been associated with some side effects. For oseltamivir, the most commonly reported side effects during research and development were nausea, vomiting, and headache. Zanamivir has been associated with allergic reactions (mouth, throat, or facial edema and skin rash), risk of spasm of the bronchi in the lungs, sinusitis, dizziness, and ear/nose/throat infections. For peramivir, diarrhea was the most common side effect. In postmarketing reports, there have also been descriptions of serious skin reactions (oseltamivir and peramivir) and sporadic, transient neuropsychiatric events (oseltamivir, peramivir, and zanamivir).

Luckily, the neuraminidase inhibitors work against both influenza A and B strains, although they are known to work more strongly against influenza A. In early studies, when oseltamivir was given a day after symptoms of influenza began, viral shedding was reduced, symptoms reported by sick people were less, and there were decreased numbers of middle ear abnormalities when compared with people who had received a placebo. Zanamivir, given as late as 50 hours after infection, also demonstrated success with reduced viral shedding, decreased symptoms reported by sick people, decreased amounts of mucus, and less middle ear abnormalities. The benefits seen in those early studies were confirmed with later testing in people with uncomplicated influenza. When started within 36 hours of flu symptoms, oseltamivir resulted in a 30–40 percent reduction in the length and severity of symptoms and also decreased the number of people who suffered from prolonged coughing. The earlier the drug was given after the start of flu symptoms, the quicker people returned to work or other normal activities. Zanamivir, when given early in the course of symptoms, also showed fewer days of symptoms and an earlier return to normal activities. Early administration also reduced the use of antibiotics and number of hospitalizations.

Historically, resistance has not been as big an issue for the NA inhibitors. However, a small increase in the number of influenza viruses resistant to oseltamivir has more recently been observed in the United States.

Endonuclease Inhibitors

A new medication for the treatment of acute uncomplicated influenza was approved by the FDA in October 2018. This medication, called baloxavir marboxil, is unique in that it is the first antiviral targeting influenza via a new mechanism of action given approval in almost 20 years. Normally, the influenza virus "steals" a short string of the host cell's RNA and attaches it to its own RNA, tricking the host cell into duplicating it; this process is known as cap snatching. Baloxavir works by binding to one of two endonuclease (an enzyme that breaks down a nucleotide chain) sites, which blocks the cap snatching. Baloxavir is given as a single oral dose to people 12 years or older who have been sick with flu symptoms for less than 48 hours; it works against both influenza A and influenza B. It is not yet clear if dose reductions might be needed for people with kidney impairment or severe liver disease.

Data documented during the research and development of baloxavir showed that it reduced the duration of influenza symptoms by more than one day, offered similar benefits as oseltamivir, and reduced the length of time that the influenza virus was shed by sick people. It appears to work against a wide range of influenza viruses, including strains that have already become resistant to oseltamivir and avian strains such as H7N9 and H5N1. Baloxavir has been noted to be generally well tolerated, and it seems to have less adverse events than oseltamivir. The most commonly reported side effects have been diarrhea, bronchitis, nasopharyngitis, headache, and nausea.

In the trials leading up to the approval of baloxavir, resistance ranged from approximately 0 to 44 percent with the higher resistance rates primarily observed in studies of children and among patients infected with the H3N2 strain of influenza A. Since baloxavir is still new, close monitoring will be needed to identify risks for emerging resistance during treatment. More studies will also need to be done to see if baloxavir will be helpful for young children and if it will be of benefit to severely ill or hospitalized patients.

6

Long-Term Prognosis and Potential Complications

Influenza is a respiratory infection with a tendency to cause marked systemic symptoms due to activation of the host's immune cascade. While for many of us the infection is short-lived, for others the infection can overwhelm the body's defenses or even cause trouble in organ systems beyond the lungs. And for an unfortunate number of people, it can even result in death.

BURDENS OF ILLNESS AND RISK OF DEATH

Every year, approximately 10–20 percent of the world's population is infected with influenza and 3–5 million hospitalizations result from the flu. As you can imagine, the costs related to seasonal influenza infections are simply enormous. While it is probably obvious that there is a considerable burden on the health system given the number of doctor visits and hospitalizations related to the flu, it is perhaps less well known that influenza is responsible for a substantial economic burden related to more than just those direct medical costs; indirect costs, such as absenteeism from work, are exorbitant as well. One study published in 2018 set out to define the economic burden of seasonal influenza in the United States. By evaluating estimates of age-specific outcomes attributed to influenza, the researchers found that the average annual total economic burden of influenza to the health care system and society was $11.2 billion; of this total, $3.2 billion were thought to be related to direct medical costs, but indirect costs related to productivity loss were $8 billion.

Given these numbers, it is certainly evident that the societal economic burden of seasonal influenza is impressive. What then are the burdens of influenza on you as an individual? Here's a look at how getting the flu might affect you:

Financial Cost

If you get infected with the flu, you may decide to see a doctor. You'll need to pay for the visit and for any testing the doctor decides is necessary. If you have insurance, your financial obligation might be limited to a copay; if you don't have insurance, the costs of the visit and testing could be more burdensome. If you are prescribed an antiviral medication, a course could cost more than $100 for five days of treatment if you don't have insurance. Over-the-counter medications to target some of your flu symptoms will add to your expenses. Since the flu can make you feel ill and is contagious, you'll probably need to miss school or work. In the case of absence from work, you could be subject to lost income if you don't have paid sick leave. If you miss school, you might have consequences related to your grades, scholarships, sports, or other commitments. If you develop a complication of the influenza infection and require hospitalization, you'll be required to pay your portion of the hospital bill; this can amount to thousands of dollars, even with insurance.

Physical Cost

If you've ever had the flu, you might recall just how miserable it can be. It is physically draining and painful, especially if you are older than 65 or younger than five years of age. If you are one of the people who suffer complications from your influenza infection, you could endure a hospitalization. While hospitalized, you might undergo additional testing that could require removal of blood for labs or exposure to radiation for imaging. If your breathing became precarious, you might need intubation so that you can be hooked to a breathing machine for mechanical ventilation. If critically ill, you could need insertion of catheters or tubes into veins, arteries, or the urinary tract and rectum. You might be given antiviral medications or antibiotics, which have risks of side effects or allergic reactions. If organs beyond your lungs begin to fail, you could even need lifesaving measures such dialysis.

Emotional Cost

Being sick with the flu can promote developmental regression, which means that we can all feel and act younger than our actual age when ill. Evidence suggests that children and adolescents with the flu will experience worsening mood and anxiety during the infection, especially if they already have preexisting psychiatric syndromes. If you were so sick with the flu that you required hospitalization, there can be psychological trauma associated with that admission, especially if you were in the critical care unit. In addition, mental instability has been described as being a potential consequence of surviving influenza infection. Mental health effects have ranged from depression and other mood disturbances to insomnia and psychosis. If you happened to be female and pregnant when you became ill with the flu, some studies have suggested that your baby might even be at risk for bipolar disorder or psychotic disorders such as schizophrenia.

These individual burdens from influenza are scary enough, but perhaps the most worrisome take-home point regarding the flu is that it still kills people, year after year. *A lot of people.* Seasonal influenza-related deaths are those that occur in people for whom influenza infection was likely a contributor to the cause of death. Though the CDC estimates the number of deaths for each influenza season, the count is not exact. There are a number of different reasons for this: (a) states are not required to report individual flu illness or deaths for people older than 18 years of age; (b) influenza is infrequently listed on death certificates of people who die from flu-related complications; (c) many flu-related deaths occur one or two weeks after the initial infection; and (d) most people who die from flu-related complications are not tested for the flu. So, how many influenza-related deaths related to seasonal influenza have been reported in recent years? For adults, from the 2010–2011 flu season to the 2017–2018 flu season, the CDC estimates that influenza-associated deaths in the United States ranged from a low of 12,000 to a high of 79,000 (during the 2017–2018 season). For children younger than 18, influenza-associated deaths estimated by the CDC since 2010 range from 37 to about 1200 (during the 2012–2013 season).

One question that always comes to mind when reviewing the death rates for influenza is how many flu-associated deaths might have occurred in people who were not vaccinated. Unfortunately, since flu-related deaths in adults are not a reported condition, the exact number is not available in that population. However, flu-associated death in children is a nationally notifiable condition, so data is provided to the CDC, including demographic information, flu laboratory test results, clinical information, and vaccine history. During past seasons, approximately 80 percent of the flu-associated deaths in children have occurred in children who were *not vaccinated.*

COMPLICATIONS BEYOND THE LUNGS

By reviewing case reports, epidemiological investigations, and autopsy studies, researchers have been able to better define the extrapulmonary complications of infection with influenza. It is thought that either unique viral pathogenesis (e.g., the newer avian A[H5N1] strain) or human host factors (such as age, comorbidities, genetic predisposition), or both, might cause such symptoms beyond the lungs to occur. Many of the extrapulmonary complications are associated with the acute phase of the infection and might be the reason that people seek medical attention. Some, however, may follow influenza infection by weeks to months. Some people who are infected with influenza can even have more than one extrapulmonary manifestation at the same time.

Cardiovascular Complications

During influenza epidemics, there is an increase in cardiovascular (heart and blood vessel) complications leading to death, and some of the heart and vascular conditions that are exacerbated during infection with the flu include myocarditis and/or pericarditis, worsening heart failure, heart attacks, and stroke. *Myocarditis* is a medical term for inflammation of the heart muscle, while pericarditis describes inflammation of the lining (pericardium) of the heart. Myocarditis is the most commonly described cardiac complication related to influenza, and it has been reported in approximately 0.4–13 percent of hospitalized patients known to have the flu. However, it is possible that this complication is underreported, as pathological findings of myocarditis have been found in 30–50 percent of flu patients at autopsy despite no diagnosed cardiac issues prior to death. Interestingly, myocarditis related to influenza often occurs in the absence of more severe respiratory complications. It is not entirely understood why influenza infection causes myocarditis in some people. Because evidence of the flu virus can be found in biopsies of heart muscle or in fluid surrounding the heart, there is a suggestion that direct viral invasion may be an explanation. On the other hand, the increased incidence of myocarditis in people who have more severe infection could suggest an exaggerated immune response as the cause. Of the cases of influenza-associated myocarditis that have been reported in the literature, 52 percent occurred in men and 68 percent occurred in patients under 40 years of age. It has been described as a consequence of both influenza A and influenza B.

An appreciation for the symptoms of myocarditis in people infected with influenza, and early recognition by medical providers who can initiate appropriate cardiac care, is critical since risk of death due to this cardiac complication has been estimated to be 23 percent in some studies. The majority of people with myocarditis experience acute symptoms that suggest cardiac dysfunction, such as chest pain, shortness of breath, loss of consciousness, low blood pressure, and abnormal heart rate. These symptoms are most likely to occur between days 4 and 7 following viral infection. The severity of symptoms is variable and can range from completely asymptomatic to severe; there is some suggestion that a significant proportion of people with influenza may have completely unrecognized heart injury. The outcomes of influenza-associated myocarditis can include heart failure, abnormal heart rhythms (arrhythmias), collection of fluid surrounding the heart (known as a pericardial effusion), and a phenomenon called cardiac tamponade (compression of the heart due to the accumulation of fluid in the pericardial sac). Heart failure is the most common consequence.

Heart failure has also been seen in patients who have influenza without evidence of myocarditis. In one study reviewing 124 patients hospitalized with the flu, a quarter of them had diagnostic evaluation of the heart with 25 percent of those studied showing signs of heart failure. Luckily, the majority of those patients showed at least some improvement in their heart function within three weeks of infection. Other studies have shown that right-sided heart failure was more common than left-sided heart failure in patients admitted to the ICU with influenza A, and it was more likely to be found in patients with ARDS.

Large studies in Russia, the United States, the United Kingdom, and Hong Kong have shown a relationship between influenza virus circulation and an increase in hospitalizations and death from ischemic heart disease. Rates of a first heart attack have been shown to be highest in the first three days following an acute respiratory infection like the flu. Another study of 600 patients in the Veterans Administration system found that a quarter of patients who tested positive for influenza had acute cardiac injury (and 50 percent of these injuries were true heart attacks). It is thought that influenza-associated ischemic heart disease is driven by inflammation and stimulation of procoagulant effects.

Similar to ischemic cardiac complications, the risk of stroke is significantly increased in the days after a respiratory tract infection. However, cases of ischemic stroke in the setting of influenza have only been rarely reported.

Central Nervous System Complications

There are a number of neurological conditions that have been described in conjunction with influenza infection, including influenza-associated encephalopathy/encephalitis (IAE), post-influenza encephalitis, Guillain-Barré syndrome, and Parkinsonian symptoms. IAE is a rapidly progressive process characterized by an impaired level of consciousness developing within a few days of influenza infection. Within the umbrella of IAE, several distinct clinical syndromes have been described, including the following:

- Acute necrotizing encephalopathy (ANE): characterized by multiple brain lesions frequently involving the thalami
- Acute encephalopathy with biphasic seizures and late reduced diffusion (AESD): biphasic course associated with febrile seizures and subcortical white matter lesions on MRI
- Mild encephalitis with reversible splenial lesions (MERS): milder course with lesions of the splenium of the corpus callosum
- Posterior reversible encephalopathy syndrome (PRES): areas of edema on MRI occurring days to weeks after initial viral symptoms
- Acute hemorrhagic leukoencephalopathy (AHLE): rapid demyelination and inflammation of the white matter

IAE is more frequently recognized and reported in children, but the incidence has been reported to be up to 4 percent in hospitalized adults. In reports of IAE, men seem to be more affected than women and patients ranged from 20 to 86 years of age. Symptoms usually appeared early within the first week of viral illness with the neurological symptoms being the reason the people sought medical attention in 80 percent of the cases. Nearly all patients had decreased consciousness and over a third had witnessed seizure activity. Fortunately, 79 percent of patients with IAE survived, but a quarter had residual neurological deficits. Both influenza A and influenza B strains have been implicated. Post-influenza encephalopathy is the development of neurological symptoms after resolution of the respiratory illness (usually within about three weeks of diagnosis).

Symptoms described in people with this complication have included altered mentation, seizures, involuntary movements, and blindness. It is not clear why some people suffer from IAE or post-influenza encephalopathy. Evidence of the influenza virus has been found in brain tissue and cerebral spinal fluid, which might suggest direct invasion of the virus into the central nervous system. People with IAE also seem to experience higher likelihood of both liver and kidney dysfunction, raising concern for a component of metabolic encephalopathy rather than direct viral-induced central nervous system effect. Immune-mediated effects may also be possible. A genetic predisposition has also been suggested due to a higher incidence in East Asian populations.

Guillain-Barré syndrome (GBS) is an immune-mediated polyneuropathy in which the body's own immune system attacks the nerves. Named after the French neurologists George Guillain (1876–1951) and Jean Alexander Barré (1880–1967), GBS is thought to be triggered by an infectious agent, such as the influenza virus, with onset of symptoms within two to six weeks of infection. GBS is characterized by varying degrees of muscle weakness and abnormalities in sensation that first starts in the legs and, over time, may progress to the upper body and arms, eventually causing full paralysis, loss of deep tendon reflexes, and a need for total care and support. If the paralysis ascends to the level of the diaphragm and the nerves that influence respiration, patients may even require breathing assistance with a mechanical ventilator. GBS is a rare complication of influenza, and it isn't clear who may be at risk for development of GBS; unfortunately, this makes any attempt to prevent GBS difficult. Treatment for GBS is mostly supportive in nature because the disorder will often improve over time and patients may have a complete recovery. In some people, however, residual neurological deficits persist even after the acute illness has passed; rarely, some people with GBS die. Newer treatments for GBS include plasmapheresis, where the plasma from the sick person is removed and replaced with healthy donor plasma or infusion of high-dose immunoglobulins (antibodies). Two other neuro-inflammatory diseases related to GBS have been attributed to the flu: acute disseminated encephalomyelitis (ADEM) and transverse myelitis. ADEM affects both the brain and spine, while transverse myelitis involves the spinal cord along a cross section, often resulting in paralysis below the level of involvement.

Narcolepsy is a disorder characterized by excessive daytime sleepiness with nighttime disturbance, and it can be associated with the sudden loss of muscle tone (cataplexy). Upper respiratory infections like influenza have been linked to this disease. One analysis of 629 patients in China demonstrated a threefold increase in the incidence of narcolepsy after the 2009 H1N1 influenza pandemic. Encephalitis lethargica (EL) is a neuropsychiatric disorder characterized by sleep disturbances, lethargy, and movement disturbances. It was first described during the 1918 influenza pandemic, so it was thought to be caused by the flu. This was not proven by studies of brain tissue, however. Sporadic cases of EL have since been described, often following pharyngitis, but the relationship to influenza remains unclear.

Conjunctivitis and Other Ocular Complications

Influenza can cause eye problems, which is thought to be due to direct invasion by the virus into the conjunctiva (mucous membrane that lines the eyelids and eye). This most commonly results in conjunctivitis (inflammation of the conjunctiva), although involvement of the retina, abnormal fluid collection, and inflammation along the optic nerve have also been described. While conjunctivitis is usually short-lived and self-limited, these other complications may require treatments such as steroids and vision can be compromised. The avian influenza H7N7 strain seems to have a particular predilection for the conjunctival epithelium, and isolated conjunctivitis has been described in people infected with this strain of flu. During an outbreak of this influenza strain in the Netherlands, 91 percent of patients had conjunctivitis as their only symptom.

Hematological Complications

A variety of hematological complications have been associated with influenza, including blood clots and several other complicated diagnoses (thrombotic thrombocytopenic purpura or TTP, hemolytic-uremic syndrome or HUS, and hemophagocytic syndrome or HPS). There is a bit of conflicting evidence about the risk of blood clots in the setting of influenza infection. Some studies have suggested that there has been a higher incidence of pulmonary blood clots in people with the flu compared to other critically ill patients, but some studies have suggested otherwise. TTP and HUS are overlapping syndromes that are characterized by a specific type of anemia, low platelets, acute kidney injury, and neurological abnormalities; these have only rarely been associated with influenza infection. HPS is a clinical condition in which uncontrolled destruction of platelets, erythrocytes, and lymphocytes occurs due to activated macrophages and histiocytes in the setting of increased secretion of cytokines. Though this has not frequently been reported in association with influenza, there is concern that it might be underappreciated; one post-mortem review of six patients who died of influenza A(H5N1) infection had evidence of HPS on autopsy.

Kidney Complications

There are a number of kidney issues that can occur in the setting of influenza infection, including acute kidney injury and other more complicated diagnoses (acute glomerulonephritis, minimal change disease, and acute tubulointerstitial nephritis). Acute kidney injury has been observed in 18–66 percent of people with influenza who have been admitted to an intensive care unit, and the degree of injury can be variable with regard to severity; as many as 22 percent of people may proceed to dialysis. Some risk factors for the development of kidney injury in people infected with influenza include obesity, presence of chronic kidney disease prior to illness, older age, and increased severity of illness at time of admission to the hospital. It is thought that the cause of kidney injury in influenza infection could be due to a number of factors such as decreased kidney perfusion and direct viral injury.

Liver Complications

Fortunately, complications of the liver from influenza infection are only rarely reported. When it does occur, there is some suggestion that it may be related to specific flu strains. For example, studies have shown that greater proportions of people with influenza A(H1N1)pdm09 had evidence of elevated liver enzymes when compared to patients infected with the regular seasonal flu strain in 2008. A similar finding has been reported in people who were infected with A(H5N1) and A(H7N9). Also, influenza has been implicated as a trigger for development of organ rejection in people who previously underwent liver transplantation. Viral invasion into liver cells has not been reliably demonstrated, although viral particles have been found and influenza has been cultured from liver samples. It is possible that the liver may suffer during an overall systemic immune response during influenza infection or that the liver was troubled by medications that were administered during the illness.

Reye's syndrome can occur several days after a respiratory illness such as influenza and usually manifests as a combination of confusion and fatty infiltration of the liver. The most frequent laboratory abnormality seen in Reye's syndrome is elevation of ammonia in the blood. This syndrome has been connected with influenza B more frequently than with influenza A. Historically, Reye's syndrome was most strongly associated with children who were given aspirin to treat fever caused by influenza or other viruses. The incidence of Reye's syndrome has decreased significantly now that pediatricians have educated parents about the risks of aspirin use in children who are sick with respiratory infections.

Myositis and Rhabdomyolysis

It is not at all uncommon for patients who are sick with the flu to have muscle aches or myalgias. More rarely seen, however, is myositis (inflammation of the muscles) leading to rhabdomyolysis, which is the destruction of muscle tissue with release of the breakdown products into the bloodstream; this, in turn, can sometimes be a factor that leads to acute kidney injury. In cases of virus-associated rhabdomyolysis, influenza is the most commonly found agent.

Most cases of myositis occur about 72 hours after identification of influenza infection, with the great majority of people reporting symptoms within one week of the onset of respiratory symptoms. Usually, the calf muscles are involved, but other muscle groups can be affected at the same time. Symptoms can be severe enough to prevent people from walking normally. Myositis has been most commonly reported in children, and in boys more than girls. More rarely, it can occur in adults. In most cases, the symptoms resolve in about three days, although a small number of people experience symptoms for weeks.

The diagnosis of rhabdomyolysis is made by measurement of a muscle enzyme known as creatine phosphokinase (CK) in the blood. A higher degree of elevation of this enzyme has been associated with worse outcomes. People who have elevated CK levels during influenza infection are more likely to need help with breathing via a mechanical ventilator for a longer time, and they often have a longer intensive care unit stay. Rhabdomyolysis can lead to kidney failure for a variety of reasons (tubules can become obstructed with excess myoglobin, direct tubular injury, or constriction of the blood vessels in the kidneys). Some people even progress to kidney failure that is severe enough to require dialysis.

Toxic Shock Syndrome

As has been mentioned previously, *Staphylococcus aureus* is a bacterium that can cause secondary infection in people who have become sick with the flu. Some people who are infected with this organism can go on to develop toxic shock syndrome (TSS). The influenza virus is thought to actually change the replication characteristics of toxin-producing strains of *Staphylococcus aureus*. When these toxins are released into the system, severe consequences can occur, including:

- high fever;
- drop in blood pressure that doesn't respond to fluid resuscitation;
- redness of the eyes, lips, tongue, and throat;

- rash resembling sunburn, even on the palms and soles;
- nausea, vomiting, and diarrhea;
- headache, confusion, or even seizures; and
- muscle aches.

The treatment for TSS is hospitalization, antibiotics to target the *Staphylococcal* bacterium, blood pressure support, and relief for any other symptoms. Occasionally, the marked decrease in blood pressure and ongoing toxin production can lead to kidney failure, and patients need to proceed to dialysis. Rarely, the symptoms of TSS become overwhelming and death can occur.

7

Effects on Family and Friends

Most of us have been sick with an illness that we thought was likely the flu, and most of us have considered it to be a miserable infection to experience personally. It's not uncommon to question how we might have managed to come down with influenza. Did we catch it when our colleague at work sneezed without covering his nose and mouth? Did our toddler bring it home from day care? Was it during our flight home from our European vacation that we were exposed? As we ponder those questions, it is inevitable that we might also consider how our infection could spread to our family or friends and what impact influenza might have on their lives and ours.

THE SPREAD OF INFLUENZA

The flu virus is primarily spread from person to person in one of two ways. First, people who are infected with influenza can release small virus-containing droplets into the air when they cough, sneeze, or talk. These droplets can land in mouths or noses, or be breathed in, by people who are around them (even up to six feet away!), and then the virus can infect the respiratory tract of its new host. Another way that influenza is spread from person to person is through contaminated respiratory secretions on hands and other surfaces; these secretions can be spread by hands to other people, especially if the hands come in contact with the mouth, nose, or eyes. The influenza virus is pretty hardy: it can survive for up to an hour in the air in enclosed environments. On hard surfaces such as stainless steel and plastic, the influenza virus can survive for more than eight hours, and it can be transmitted for up to five minutes on hands after it has transferred from another surface.

One factor that likely contributes to the spread of influenza is that the virus can be found in respiratory secretions before a person realizes they are sick or before any symptoms have become evident to others around them. Most healthy adults can infect others for at least a day before they experience any symptoms at all, and they continue to be infectious to others for days after becoming sick. They are most contagious, though, for the first three to four days of their illness. Young children are usually considered to be the greatest spreaders of the flu because they produce more viruses in their respiratory tract than do adolescents and adults. In addition, young children are less likely to practice good hygiene that would inhibit the spread of the virus, such as good cough and sneeze etiquette and frequent handwashing. They also are often contagious for a longer period of time than adolescents and adults, and they can spread the flu to others for more than seven days after becoming ill. It is children who drive the local spread of influenza within schools, households, and cities in general.

As you know, influenza is a seasonal virus, and there are factors that have been suggested to account for increased spread of the virus during the winter months, including

- indoor crowding during cold weather;
- seasonal fluctuations in host immune responses;
- relative humidity (particularly when normal humid air turns dry);
- low temperatures; and
- UV radiation levels.

It is known that seasons with higher rates of death from influenza are associated with higher disease transmission and more rapid spread than milder seasons. It's also clear that influenza, while still a seasonal virus, might more easily and rapidly spread in the face of our planet's climate changes and our more global population. Historically, as we explored in chapter 2, the spread of influenza was linked to our participation in warfare with the movement of troops. In more contemporary times, it is air travel that is considered to be a primary factor in the global spread of infectious agents such as influenza.

Narrowing the view to the United States, it has been shown that there has previously been a tendency for the influenza season to start in California more often than in any other state. One reason for this is that California is more heavily populated. However, another key factor might include workflow (rates of movement of people to and from their workplaces), which has been shown to be a key predictor of regional influenza spread. A more recent study looked at the effect of employment rates on the spread of the flu. Researchers found that an increase of only one percentage point in the employment rate increased the number of flu-related outpatient doctor visits by 19 percent; these effects were most highly pronounced in the retail and health care sectors due to high levels of interpersonal contact. Labor market-based activities, such as public transportation, carpools, working in offices, putting children in day care, and having frequent contact with the public, are all suggested to contribute to the spread of the flu.

Another recent investigation using several large datasets describing health care visits, geographic movements, and demographics of more than 150 million people over nine years has allowed the creation of models that predict the spread of influenza through the United States. These models have suggested that seasonal flu outbreaks will tend to originate in warm, humid areas of the south and southeastern United States (counties on the coasts near the Gulf of Mexico or the Atlantic Ocean) and then move northward, away from the coasts. Interestingly, some of the factors that contributed to this proposed pathway of spread were the following:

- An unusually high level of social connectivity in the southern United States (the number of close friends, close friends who are neighbors, and communities of people who all, or mostly all, know each other is much higher in the South than in the country at large)
- A unique combination of weather and demographic factors
- The collective movement of people over short distances (travel from the coastlines inward to the center of the continent)

Further discussion about the global spread of influenza can be found in chapters 9 and 10.

DEALING WITH ILLNESS IN A LOVED ONE

Thankfully, for many people, influenza is a fairly short and self-limited illness with few long-standing consequences. Most of us already know enough about the flu to adopt good practices in the setting of illness: we stay home from work or school, we remain in bed and sleep more, and we use over-the-counter cold medications and pain alleviators in order to feel better. Because it is so important to treat those with the flu appropriately and to try to limit the spread of infection, the CDC has published brochures specifically designed to help people care for themselves and others who might be suffering from influenza. Remember that the first step for all of us is to avoid getting the flu by following these recommendations:

- Get the flu vaccine.
- Cover your nose and mouth with a tissue when you cough or sneeze. Throw the tissue in the trash after you use it. If you don't have a tissue available, cough into your upper arm.
- Wash your hands often with soap and water. If soap and water aren't readily available, use an alcohol-based hand rub.
- Avoid touching your eyes, nose, and mouth.
- Try to limit your contact with other sick people.

If, by chance, you do become ill, you should recognize the symptoms of the flu, including fever and/or chills, cough, sore throat, runny or stuffy nose, muscle or body aches, headache, tiredness, and possible nausea with vomiting. If you think the symptoms are consistent with the flu, you should stay at home except to get medical care or other necessities. If you think someone you love has the flu, there are things you can do to help minimize the spread of the infection, offer the sick person some relief from their suffering, and, hopefully, minimize complications. Your loved one with the flu should also be encouraged to stay at home except to get medical care or other necessities until at least 24 hours after they are free of a fever without having taken any antipyretics (such as acetaminophen or ibuprofen). A sick person can find relief in staying in bed to get restorative sleep, being near a private restroom should they need it frequently, and having access to medications and hydration. Also, they are less likely to infect others if they remain at home.

The Sick Room

While at home, it is best to make a separate sick room for the person who is ill; this is another way to limit the spread of the flu to others in the home or immediate environment. If there is more than one bathroom available, try to have the sick person consistently use just one of them; people who are well should use a separate bathroom. It is also helpful to give the sick person their own drinking glass, washcloth, and towel to use. Helpful items to keep in the sick room might include tissues, trash can (with a lid and a plastic liner, if at all possible), alcohol-based hand sanitizer, a cooler or pitcher with ice and drinks, a cup with a straw (or a squeeze bottle) to help with keeping hydrated, a thermometer, a humidifier (a machine that puts tiny drops of water into the air, allowing for extra moisture that can make it easier to breathe), and facemasks that the sick person can wear when they leave the sick room or are around other people. Medications can also be stored in the sick room, but they should be out of the reach of children. It can be helpful to have the names of the medications and the dosing schedules written down for reference (remember that children aged 18 or younger should not be given products with aspirin in them due to the risk of Reye's syndrome).

It is best to choose one primary caregiver to enter the room and to prevent other visitors from entering the room as much as possible. When considering who should be the caregiver, remember that empathy is an important characteristic. Empathy, simply put, is the ability to recognize and understand the feelings, thoughts, and experiences of someone else, and this trait can be particularly helpful when caring for a sick loved one. Medical studies have actually shown that patients who were under the care of providers who were found to be highly empathetic were sick nearly a day less and had better levels of certain immune system markers than patients with less empathetic providers. Good empathetic care of a sick loved one might include

- making the sick person feel comfortable and at ease by keeping them warm;
- making sure they have a source of entertainment, such as books, TV, movies, or video games;
- keeping tissues (and medications, if an adult) within reach;
- offering enough food and liquids;
- listening actively without interrupting;
- maintaining attentiveness;
- taking care of chores or errands that the sick person can't get done;
- being positive with a focus on recovery; and
- explaining care clearly while allowing the loved one to express their preferences.

If other people do enter the sick room, they should stay at least six feet away from the sick person. The sick person should cover their nose and mouth with a tissue when they cough and sneeze (and then throw used tissues directly in the trash can), and the air in the sick room should be kept clean by opening windows or using a fan to keep fresh air flowing if the weather permits it. Caregivers should avoid being face-to-face with the sick person, and it is best to spend the least amount of time possible in close contact with the sick person. When holding sick children, caregivers should place the child's chin on their shoulder (to help direct the cough away from their own nose and mouth). Caregivers should wash their hands often (especially after touching the sick person or handling their tissues or laundry), and if soap and water aren't available, an alcohol-based hand rub should be used frequently. Sick people with the flu should drink extra fluids to keep from getting dehydrated. It is okay to continue to nurse or bottle feed a baby with the flu. For children and adults, any caffeinated colas, tea, and coffee should be avoided, as should alcoholic beverages. In addition to water, mild broth or sport drinks with low sugar content can be consumed. If the sick person is too ill to drink from a cup, use a squeeze bottle or straw; ice chips or frozen ice pops can also be used to help prevent dehydration. The sick room should be cleaned each day. For hard surfaces like doorknobs, bedside tables, bathroom sinks, toilets, counters, phones, and toys, cleaning with water and dish soap is fine; other common household cleaners that kill germs also can be used. Bed sheets and towels should be cleaned with normal laundry soap and a hot dryer setting. All dirty laundry should be held away from the face and body, and hands should be washed right after touching dirty laundry. Dishes can be washed with normal dish soap or in a dishwasher. See Table 7.1 for further influenza care and management recommendations.

Table 7.1 Influenza Care and Management

	Dos	**Don'ts**
Medications	Read the label and take only the dosing recommended.	Never give aspirin to children age 18 or under if they have the flu.
	Talk to your doctor if you are pregnant before taking medications	Don't drink alcohol and take medicine.
	Store medications out of the reach of children.	Don't give cough or cold medicines to children younger than four years of age.
Fever	Place a cool, damp washcloth on the forehead; wash arms and body with a cool cloth.	Don't take a very hot bath (can consider a slightly warm bath).
	Use medicines that list acetaminophen or ibuprofen on the labels.	Don't exceed the dosing limits of antipyretics.
Cough	Ask the pharmacist about which medications might be best.	Don't give cough medicine to any child less than four years of age.

Table 7.1 Influenza Care and Management (*Continued*)

	Dos	Don'ts
	Set up a humidifier.	Don't forget to clean the humidifier frequently.
	Offer adults a cough drop or hard candy to soothe the throat and lessen the urge to cough.	Don't give children under the age of four a cough drop or hard candy (they can be at risk for choking).
Sore Throat	Offer acetaminophen or ibuprofen for the pain.	Don't offer saltwater gargle (one cup of warm water plus one teaspoon of salt) to children less than six years of age.
	Consider use of either warm liquids (broth, caffeine-free tea, or warm water with honey) or cold treats (ice chips or frozen ice pops) to soothe the throat and to help get fluids into the body.	Avoid cigarette smoke and cleaning products that can irritate the throat.
Chills and Aches/Pains	Offer a light blanket for chills.	Don't use heated blankets or pads in one area for an extended period due to risk of burns.
	Use acetaminophen or ibuprofen to lessen pain.	Don't overexert your muscles or engage in high-impact activity if they are hurting.
	Place a warm washcloth on the face to ease sinus pains caused by congestion.	
Stomach Problems	Stick with plain foods that are easy on the stomach. One example is the BRAT diet: bananas, rice, applesauce, and toast.	Don't eat spicy foods, high fat or fried foods, or acidic foods until the stomach can handle them.
	Try to drink mostly clear liquids.	Don't drink only sugary sports drinks or soda.
	Consider medicines for adults that might help lessen loose stools.	

Emergency Warning Signs

Caregivers need to recognize that there are emergency warning signs during influenza infection that should prompt a sick person to seek medical care urgently. According to the CDC, in infants and children, these emergency warning signs include

- fast breathing or trouble breathing;
- bluish skin color;
- not drinking enough fluids and/or not being able to eat;
- not waking up and/or not interacting;
- being so irritable that the child does not want to be held;
- return of fever and worse cough after an initial period of improvement;
- fever with a rash (and any child younger than three months with a fever should be seen by a doctor);
- having no tears when crying; and
- having significantly fewer wet diapers than normal.

For adolescents and adults, the emergency warning signs during influenza infection that warrant urgent medical attention per the CDC include

- notable difficulty breathing or shortness of breath;
- pain or pressure in the chest or abdomen;
- sudden dizziness;
- confusion;
- severe or persistent vomiting; and
- flu-like symptoms that improve but then return with fever and worse cough.

Hospitalization

Sometimes, a person is so sick with influenza that they require hospitalization. Though a family member won't be acting as a primary caregiver in this circumstance, there are a number of guidelines that focus on being a good hospital visitor:

- Before you visit a patient in the hospital, check with other family members or the nursing staff to determine if the patient is feeling well enough to have visitors and when it might be the best time to visit.
- Always check in at the front desk when arriving on the patient's floor to see if the patient is available for a visit. Showing up unannounced at

the room can be a disturbance if the patient is sleeping, undergoing a bath, or away for testing. In addition, many facilities limit the number of visitors in a room at a time.

- Follow the hospital's policies for visiting hours, especially in the intensive care unit. It is best to avoid visitation during a change of shift (often between seven and eight in the morning and again between three and four in the late afternoon). Of note, the busiest time of day for medical staff and nurses is between 6:00 a.m. and 11:00 a.m. when medications are being given, baths are underway, and labs are being drawn, so it can sometimes be difficult to get patient updates then.
- Do not visit a patient in the hospital if you are sick. You don't want to spread any germs to people in the hospital, so consider sending a card or calling the patient on the phone instead.
- Always follow the infection control protocols of the facility, including using hand sanitizer upon entering and leaving the patient's room and/or wearing a mask if it is required. Don't sit on the patient's bed and don't touch any of the equipment.
- Don't wear perfume or cologne and try not to smoke before visiting the hospital, as strong scents can trigger upset stomach or be uncomfortable to a sick patient's sense of smell.
- Don't bring food and drink. Though these gifts seem thoughtful to you, patients often have strict limitations on their diet or fluid intake, or they may be too sick to eat or drink safely. Also, you shouldn't eat from the patient's hospital tray, even if they don't finish their food, since the medical staff might be closely monitoring the patient's nutritional intake.
- Don't bring flowers or latex balloons, as many patients (or their roommates) may have allergies or sensitivities to these items. In addition, some hospital units completely forbid these items.
- Don't bring outside clothing, pillows, or blankets from home. Though these might seem comforting to the patient, hospital bedding and gowns are cleaned with strict guidelines. You also don't want to return contaminated items back to the home upon hospital discharge.
- Be aware of the patient's capabilities to enjoy company and limit your visitation time accordingly. Often, nurses recommend a maximum visit time of 15–20 minutes. If the patient keeps falling asleep during your visit, let them rest. Try to avoid loud voices and show respect for the patient's roommate, too.
- Unless it is absolutely necessary, avoid bringing children to the hospital. It can be difficult to keep kids on their best behavior in the hospital environment, which is disruptive to both patients and staff. It is also

risky for children, as they tend to play on the floor, touch contaminated items, and put things in their mouths—this puts them at risk for becoming infected, too.

- Have a relaxed and positive attitude so that the patient can focus on getting well. Try not to comment on the hospital food, question the diagnoses of the medical staff, or share stories of hospital stays that have not gone well in the past.
- Designate one spokesperson to ask the staff for updates. Be aware that medical personnel may not be authorized to answer your questions or share medical information about the patient if you are not the emergency contact, patient advocate, or power of attorney.
- Remember to take care of yourself so that you can be ready to provide attention to your loved one when they return home.

8

Prevention

While the flu is often thought of as a common and rather unassuming seasonal infection, the impressive personal, economic, and societal repercussions of influenza are anything but that. Clearly, then, the best practice would be to prevent infection with the influenza virus from ever occurring. There are some practical techniques that can help people avoid contact with the flu virus, as well as judicious use of preventative medications that might help. However, the most important measure that can lessen the burden of each influenza season and attempt to limit the consequences of a future pandemic is vaccination. Studies have shown that vaccination halves the risk for influenza-related hospitalization in adults and reduces the risk for pediatric deaths from influenza by 65 percent among healthy children and by 51 percent among children with high-risk medical conditions.

INFLUENZA VACCINES

In the United States, there are essentially two main objectives when developing and promoting vaccines for influenza: (a) to protect people against infection and its potentially devastating consequences and (b) to achieve a high vaccination rate in order to ensure protection in unvaccinated people (the concept of herd immunity). In chapter 2, the evolution of influenza vaccination research and availability was discussed in detail. In this chapter, you'll learn about the recommendations regarding timing of vaccination, the currently available vaccines for influenza, and guidance for vaccine use in particular populations.

All people who are six months of age or older and who do not have contraindications should be vaccinated against influenza *every year.* Vaccination to prevent influenza is particularly important for people who are at increased risk for severe illness and complications from influenza, as well as those who may be at increased risk for influenza-related outpatient, emergency department, or hospital visits. So, when vaccine supply is limited, those higher risk persons should take priority with regard to vaccination efforts. People at high risk include the following groups:

- All children aged 6 through 59 months
- All people aged 50 years or higher
- Adults and children who have chronic lung, heart, kidney, liver, blood, or metabolic disorders
- People who are immunocompromised due to any cause
- Women who are or will be pregnant during the flu season
- Children and adolescents between the ages of 6 months and 18 years who are receiving aspirin (or salicylate-containing mediations) and who might be at risk for experiencing Reye's syndrome after influenza infection
- Residents of nursing homes and other long-term care facilities
- American Indians and Alaska Natives
- Persons who are extremely obese

Priority for vaccination is also appropriate for people who live with and care for those who are at increased risk of influenza-related complications, as well as health care personnel.

Generally speaking, it is usually recommended that people receive their flu vaccine by the end of October. This date takes into account the unpredictability of the start of the flu season and the concerns that vaccine-induced immunity might wane over the course of a season. At this time, there is no recommendation for revaccination later in the season for people who have already undergone earlier vaccination. However, if a person was not vaccinated prior to the end of October and the flu season is still circulating in their community beyond this date, vaccination should still be offered. To avoid missed opportunities for vaccination, providers should offer flu vaccines to their patients during routine health care visits and hospitalizations. Children ages 6 months through 8 years require two doses of influenza vaccine administered a minimum of four weeks apart during their first season of vaccination for the best protection; this consideration is important when scheduling children for their shots in order to ensure that both doses are given prior to the end of October.

There are general contraindications and precautions with any type of vaccination, including the vaccine for the flu. It is not usually recommended that a person undergo vaccination if they are suffering from a moderate or severe acute illness, with or without fever. Another precaution is a history of Guillain-Barré syndrome within six weeks after receiving a previous dose of an influenza vaccine. Severe allergic reactions to vaccines, although rare, can occur (even if no such reaction has occurred with vaccination before). Any person with a history of severe allergic reaction to a previous dose of any influenza vaccine, regardless of the component suspected of being responsible for the reaction, should not receive any future influenza vaccination. Many people believe that having an egg allergy would mean they shouldn't receive the flu vaccine; however, this is actually not true. People with a history of egg allergy who have experienced hives should still receive influenza vaccine; any licensed, recommended influenza vaccine that is otherwise appropriate for the recipient's age and health status can be used. People who have reactions to eggs other than hives (e.g., swelling or breathing troubles) can also receive a licensed, recommended influenza vaccine that is otherwise appropriate for their age and health status; however, the vaccine should be administered in an inpatient or outpatient medical setting and supervised by a health care provider who is able to recognize and manage severe allergic reactions should one occur.

Should you be concerned about a reaction to any of the influenza vaccines, the first step is to call your medical provider to determine if any evaluation and/or intervention is needed. With any health problem occurring after vaccination, a report can be submitted to the Vaccine Adverse Event Reporting System (VAERS). VAERS is a national vaccine safety surveillance program run by the CDC and FDA; it was created in 1990 in response to the National Childhood Vaccine Injury Act. The main goals of VAERS are to (a) detect new, unusual, or rare adverse events that happen after vaccination, (b) monitor increases in known side effects, (c) identify potential patient risk factors for particular types of health problems related to vaccines, (d) assess the safety of newly licensed vaccines, (e) watch for unexpected or unusual patterns in adverse event reports, and (f) serve as a monitoring system in public health emergencies. Once a report is filed with VAERS, it is assigned an identification number, which can be used if additional information is necessary or if follow-up by CDC or FDA scientists is warranted. Each year, about 30,000 VAERS reports are filed; most of these (85–90 percent) are descriptions of mild side effects consistent with already known vaccine consequences such as fever, arm soreness at the injection site, or crying and irritability in infants or toddlers. The remaining reports are classified as serious, indicating that the adverse event resulted in permanent disability, hospitalization, life-threatening illness, or death (of note, these are rarely found to be caused by the vaccine). For serious cases that were not considered resolved at the time of the report, a letter is sent out a year later to check on the patient's recovery status. Anyone (doctors, nurses, and the general public) can submit a report to VAERS via an online submission form. You can also access VAERS data online through a system called VAERS WONDER.

Separate and unrelated to VAERS is the Vaccine Injury Compensation Program (VICP), which is run by the Health Resources and Services Administration. This program was created after the political and financial fallout from the 1976 Swine flu vaccination plan (see chapter 2 for details), and it compensates people whose injuries may have been caused by certain vaccines. Any individual of any age who received a vaccine covered by the program and believes they were injured as a result of that vaccination can file a petition for compensation. Seasonal influenza vaccines are included in the VICP.

Killed Virus Vaccines

Killed virus vaccines are commonly referred to as inactivated influenza vaccines or IIVs. Currently, there are three different types of IIVs: standard dose, high dose, and adjuvanted. High dose influenza vaccines contain four times the amount of antigen contained in the standard dose shots in order to create a stronger immune response, while adjuvanted vaccines include ingredients that are known to prompt a more robust immune reaction. For the 2019–2020 flu season, all standard-dose IIVs were quadrivalent, meaning they contained four different flu strains. The high-dose and adjuvanted IIVs were trivalent, containing three strains. Standard dose vaccines are available for people aged 6 months and older. The high-dose and adjuvanted vaccines are licensed for persons aged 65 years and older. The IIVs are primarily administered via an intramuscular injection, with the deltoid being the preferred site for adults and older children; infants and younger children are vaccinated in the thigh. There is an intradermal IIV available as well.

Production of IIVs is complicated and involves multiple manufacturing steps:

1. A reference laboratory (often the CDC) grows each of the selected influenza strains in combination with a strain known as PR8. PR8 is a laboratory-raised strain of influenza that is inactive and unable to replicate in humans.
2. As reassortment occurs, the resulting virus contains six of the PR8 genes, along with the HA and NA of the seasonal flu strains.

3. The new reassorted virus is incubated in embryonated hens' eggs for two to three days.
4. The allantoic fluid is harvested, and the viral particles are purified at a specific density by centrifugation in a solution of increasing density.
5. The viruses are inactivated using formaldehyde or beta-propiolactone.
6. At this point, the vaccine production can be continued in one of two ways: completion as a whole virus vaccine or as a split (or subunit) virus vaccine. In a split virus vaccine, the centrifuged viral particles are washed with a detergent or ether, and the HA and NA are purified as the other viral components are removed. The remaining vaccine production steps then include the following:
    - The concentrations are standardized by the amount of hemagglutinin that occurs.
    - The strains are tested to ensure adequate yield, purity, and potency.
    - Each of the desired strains (all produced separately) is then combined into one vaccine.
    - The content of the combined vaccine is verified.
    - The combined vaccine is packaged into syringes for distribution.

Side effects to the killed virus vaccines can include the following:

- Guillain-Barré syndrome: A rare occurrence with an annual reporting rate of 0.04 in 2002–2003 and not clearly linked to IIVs. Studies suggest that the risk of developing GBS after having the flu is higher than any potential risk of developing GBS after vaccination.
- Localized injection site reactions: Pain, redness, and swelling lasting one to two days are not uncommon (reported in 10–64 percent of people) but usually do not interfere with activity.
- Systemic side effects: Headache, fever, malaise, fainting, and myalgias can occur, but most often affect people who have had no previous exposure to the influenza viruses in the vaccine.
- Febrile seizures: They occur in young children after receiving IIVs in some influenza seasons, particularly when the vaccine is given together with other vaccines (the 13-valent pneumococcal conjugate vaccine and the diphtheria/tetanus/pertussis vaccine).

Of note, the split or subunit vaccines appear to cause fewer local reactions when administered compared to whole virus vaccines, and a single dose still produces an adequate antibody reaction in a population exposed to similar viruses. However, this is not believed to be sufficient if a new influenza strain emerges, so two doses will be required for immunity in the event of a pandemic. As demonstrated by the above manufacturing description, the inactivated or killed virus vaccines do not contain a live virus; thus, these vaccines *do not* cause infection with influenza. The specific systemic side effects that prompt people to think they caught the flu from vaccination are attributable to the immune response triggered by the vaccine.

Cell Culture–based Inactivated Vaccine

The one available cell culture–based inactivated influenza vaccine, known as ccIIV, for the 2019–2020 season had a different production technique than the IIVs: the viral strains were grown in cultured cells of mammalian origin instead of hens' eggs. This vaccine was developed to provide an alternative to the egg-based manufacturing process, eliminating concerns for those who may have egg allergies. Another potential advantage of this cell culture technology is that it may serve to hasten vaccine production, both because the cells used in this process are kept frozen to be readily available and because there are no limitations imposed by the egg supply; this could prove helpful in the setting of a pandemic concern when timely vaccination production is of utmost concern. The ccIIV has the added benefit of potentially offering better protection than IIVs because influenza viruses grown in eggs undergo some changes that cause differences between the vaccine viral strains and those circulating in the population; ccIIVs should reduce these changes and allow the vaccine to contain virus that may prompt an immune response similar to the wild-type, circulating viral strains.

The ccIIV is quadrivalent (contains four viral strains) and is indicated for use in people 18 years of age and older. It is given via intramuscular injection. The most common adverse events associated with the ccIIV are injection site pain or redness, headache, fatigue, muscle pain, and malaise.

Recombinant Vaccine

In the 2019–2020 flu season, one recombinant hemagglutinin influenza vaccine, known as RIV, was available. The RIV is solely composed of the HA proteins from the chosen circulating viral strains rather than inactivated or weakened virus. The manufacturing process for the RIV, which is the fastest of all influenza vaccines, is as follows:

1. Scientists first obtain DNA for making the HA found on the desired influenza viral strain.

2. This DNA is combined with a baculovirus (a virus that is able to infect invertebrates) that helps transport the DNA instructions for making the HA into an insect host cell.
3. Once in a host cell, the resulting recombinant virus instructs the cell to produce the HA antigen, which is grown in bulk.
4. The HA antigen is collected and purified.
5. Once all HA antigens are available, they are packaged as the recombinant flu vaccine.

Since the HA proteins are made in insect cells, the need for chicken eggs is obsolete; this, in turn, eliminates the concern for vaccine allergic reaction in those who are sensitive to eggs. This vaccine is not licensed for anyone younger than 18 years of age, and it is administered via an intramuscular injection. The most common adverse effects of the RIV include injection-site pain, headache, fatigue, and myalgias.

Live Virus Vaccine

Live virus vaccines are commonly referred to as live attenuated influenza vaccines or LAIV. Only one product in this category was available for the 2019–2020 flu season: the quadrivalent intranasal vaccine or LAIV4. This vaccine is licensed for people two years of age through 49 years of age. The LAIV4 vaccine comes as a prefilled, single-use sprayer. Half of the contents are sprayed into the first nostril while the recipient sits upright; a dose-divider clip is then removed, and the second half of the vaccine is sprayed into the other nostril. If the recipient sneezes immediately after the administration of the vaccine, the dose isn't repeated. However, if nasal congestion is present that could inhibit adequate delivery of the vaccine to the nasopharyngeal mucosa, then the vaccine administration should either be deferred until resolution of the problem or another vaccine should be administered instead.

The live virus vaccine for influenza consists of a master attenuated virus into which the HA and NA genes have been inserted. The master virus is "cold adapted," which means that it replicates at an ideal temperature of 25 degrees Celsius. Thus, in the normal human body with a temperature of 37 degrees Celsius, the virus is attenuated and unlikely to cause infection while still offering a robust immune response. LAIV4 should be used with caution in children aged five years or older with the diagnosis of asthma and in individuals who have other medical conditions that place them at increased risk for complications from influenza (chronic heart or lung disease, neurological or neuromuscular diseases, metabolic diseases such as diabetes, kidney or liver dysfunction, and hematologic disorders). LAIV4 should not be used at all in the following groups:

- Children aged two through four years who have received a diagnosis of asthma or whose parents/caregivers report that a health care provider or medical record has said that the child had wheezing or asthma within the preceding 12 months
- Children aged two through seven years receiving aspirin or other salicylates
- People who are immunocompromised due to any cause (including but not limited to medications and HIV infection)
- Close contacts and caregivers of severely immunocompromised persons who require a protected environment
- Women who are pregnant
- People who have received influenza antiviral medications within the previous 48 hours

Side effects to the live virus vaccine include (a) asthma exacerbations, which have been primarily reported in children, especially those aged 6–23 months; (b) localized symptoms related to the intranasal spray, such as runny nose and congestion, sore throat (mostly reported in adults), and headache; and (c) systemic symptoms, including fever in children, abdominal pain, vomiting, and myalgias.

MEDICATIONS USED TO PREVENT INFLUENZA

It has been shown that when properly used, antiviral medications can be quite effective in preventing infection with influenza. This preventative concept is known as chemoprophylaxis. In 2018, the Infectious Disease Society of America published an updated clinical practice guideline for influenza, which included recommendations on chemoprophylaxis. Several studies have evaluated the success of post-exposure chemoprophylaxis for household members after the flu has been diagnosed within the household. In each of these studies, the efficacy in preventing the diagnosis of flu ranged from 64 percent to 81 percent. Of note, data on the ability of post-exposure chemoprophylaxis to prevent serious complications of influenza are not available (although reductions in symptomatic cases of influenza would also be expected to reduce the risk of complications of influenza).

Antiviral drugs are most often indicated for chemoprophylaxis of influenza in the setting of institutional outbreaks. However, there are other clinical situations that might prompt consideration of chemoprophylaxis.

Decisions on whether to administer post-exposure antiviral chemoprophylaxis should take into account the nature and timing of the exposure, the exposed person's risk of developing complications from influenza, the ability to promptly change the medication's dosing to treatment level should symptoms occur, advice from public health authorities, and good clinical judgment. In addition, the decision to use antiviral chemoprophylaxis should always be weighed against the prevalence of, and potential emergence of, circulating resistant viruses and the potential for side effects from the medications.

Specific scenarios that might prompt use of chemoprophylaxis include the following:

- Adults and children three months of age and older who are at very high risk of developing complications from influenza and for whom influenza vaccination is contraindicated, unavailable, or expected to have low effectiveness (e.g., in those people who are very immunocompromised). In this group of people, the pre-exposure chemoprophylaxis needs to be started as soon as the flu is detected in the community and is continued for the duration of the local seasonal outbreak.
- Adults and children three months of age and older who have the highest risk of influenza-associated complications, such as people with recent stem cell transplants or lung transplants. In this group of people, the pre-exposure chemoprophylaxis needs to be started as soon as the flu is detected in the community and is continued for the duration of the local seasonal outbreak.
- Unvaccinated adults and children three months of age and older who are at high risk of developing complications from influenza and in whom vaccination is expected to be effective but not yet administered when influenza is detected in the community. In this group of people, the chemoprophylaxis is short term and post-exposure; it is also given in conjunction with the inactivated influenza vaccine.
- Unvaccinated adults (including health care personnel) and children three months of age and older who are in close contact with persons at high risk of developing influenza complications during periods of influenza activity when vaccination is contraindicated or unavailable and those persons who are unable to take chemoprophylaxis themselves. In this group of people, the chemoprophylaxis is post-exposure and short term.

Ideally, post-exposure chemoprophylaxis should be started as soon as possible (no later than 48 hours after exposure). It is not recommended to proceed with chemoprophylaxis if more than 48 hours have passed from the time of exposure. In a non-outbreak situation, the chemoprophylaxis is

Table 8.1 Antiviral Medications Recommended for Influenza Chemoprophylaxis

Antiviral Name	Route of Administration	Age Recommendation	Standard Dosing/ Frequency
M2 Inhibitors	No longer recommended		
Neuraminidase Inhibitors			
Oseltamivir	Oral	3 months and older	75 mg once daily for >=7 days for adolescents and adults; weight-based dosing for infants and children
Zanamivir	Inhaled	5 years and older	10 mg (two 5 mg inhalations) once daily for 7 days after last known exposure
Peramivir	Intravenous	Not recommended for chemoprophylaxis	
Endonuclease Inhibitors			
Baloxavir marboxil	Oral	Not yet recommended for chemoprophylaxis	

continued for seven days after the most recent exposure to a close contact with influenza. If symptoms occur, then the post-exposure prophylaxis should be transitioned to full-dose treatment.

Though there are three classes of antiviral medications available for treatment of influenza, only two of these classes have been recommended for use as chemoprophylaxis: M2 inhibitors and neuraminidase inhibitors. The newer class of endonuclease inhibitors have not yet been recommended for use in the prevention of influenza (see Table 8.1).

M2 Inhibitors

The M2 inhibitors, amantadine and rimantadine, were previously shown to reduce infection rates during the influenza season by 50–90 percent when used as daily prophylaxis, though postexposure prophylaxis was not quite as protective. Unfortunately, as was mentioned earlier in chapter 5, use of the M2 inhibitors is now limited due to the development of resistance, and the CDC no longer recommends use of either amantadine or rimantadine for the prevention of influenza.

Neuraminidase Inhibitors

Luckily, the neuraminidase inhibitors are still recommended for the prevention of influenza. When given at the start of an influenza outbreak, these medications reduce the risk of developing the flu by 60–90 percent. The recommended oral dose of oseltamivir for prophylaxis of influenza in infants and children is based on their weight; for adults and adolescents 13 years and older, it is recommended to give 75 mg once daily for at least seven days after close contact with an infected individual. Therapy should begin within two days of exposure. Dose adjustment is recommended for patients with kidney failure; in these patients, the dose should be reduced to 75 mg every other day or 30 mg every day. For prevention of influenza using zanamivir, the dosage is two oral inhalations at 5 mg per inhalation once daily for seven days after the last known exposure. Though it is also in the class of neuraminidase inhibitors, peramivir is not recommended for chemoprophylactic use.

TECHNIQUES TO PREVENT INFECTION

Unlike some other pathogens that can only be spread from human to human via a single route, the influenza virus can be transmitted in a number of ways, including droplets, droplet nuclei, and by contact. This means that attempts at prevention must take into account each of these modes of transmission. In addition to the use of vaccines and antiviral chemoprophylaxis, adequate prevention of influenza requires education. Many people already understand that they might catch the flu by being exposed to the sneeze or cough of an infected person. However, they may not realize that even if the infected person is wearing a mask, they can potentially still spread the virus whenever they shake hands. During the handshake, the virus can easily make its way from the infected person's hands to the hands of the exposed person, who then transmits the virus to the mucous membranes of their respiratory tract when they wipe their nose.

Both the public and health care personnel need to be aware of basic personal hygiene and everyday preventive actions to stop the spread of germs and help prevent the flu. Here are some actions recommended by the CDC:

- Though it may sound simple, it is best to avoid close contact with sick people.
- If you are sick, limit your contact with others as much as possible to keep from infecting them.

- If you are sick with a flu-like illness, stay home for at least 24 hours *after* your fever is gone without the use of fever-reducing medicine, except to get medical care or other necessities.
- Clean and disinfect surfaces and objects that may be contaminated with germs like influenza.

There are techniques that attempt to limit the spread of flu when sneezing, coughing, or touching. First, cover your nose and mouth with a tissue when you cough or sneeze. After using the tissue, throw it in the trash and then wash your hands. If you don't have a tissue, don't cover your nose and mouth with your hands—use your elbow or upper arm instead. Secondly, wash your hands often with soap and water. If soap and water are not available, use an alcohol-based hand rub. Avoid touching your eyes, nose, and mouth.

When a patient has been admitted to the hospital with influenza, every attempt to place them in a single room should be made. When this is not possible, a technique called cohorting is adopted; this places patients with similar illnesses in the same room. Isolation protocols called Standard Precautions and Droplet Precautions are utilized for rooms of patients diagnosed with (or suspected of having) influenza. With Standard Precautions, all visitors who are ill are not allowed to enter the room, and visitors who do enter the room are required to cleanse their hands on their way into the room and on their way out of the room. With Droplet Precautions, all people entering the room are required to wear a face mask in addition to handwashing. Upon leaving the room, visitors throw away the face mask and again clean their hands before entering the hallway. Standard Precautions remain in place for every patient for the duration of their hospital stay. The Droplet Precautions remain in place for the initial five to seven days of illness with the flu, although a longer duration of isolation may be considered in some patients (such as those who are immunocompromised) because they can be infectious for longer periods of time.

9

Issues and Controversies

Influenza, despite being a rather simple viral particle in structure, is difficult to prevent, treat, and manage because of its ability to mutate, to jump species, and to cause significant disease with impressive societal and economic consequences year after year. Compounding these worries are a number of issues and controversies related to the global movement of humans (and our ongoing influence on the environment and other species) and the influenza vaccine.

THE GLOBAL SPREAD OF DISEASE

For much of our human history, populations have been relatively isolated from each other. It has only been in recent times that both travel and exposure have allowed extensive contact between people, plants, and animals. In that same timeline, our world population has blossomed; estimates suggest that since the influenza pandemic of 1918, the human population has increased threefold, and in the United States, international tourist arrivals have increased 35-fold. As the number of humans increases, so does the population of animals (particularly those used by humans for food). More and more animals such as dogs, chickens, pigs, cows, and rats live in and near human habitats. As an example, at the time of the 1968 influenza pandemic, the pig population in China was 5.2 million and the poultry population was 12.3 million; however, by 2005, the pig population had increased 100-fold to 503 million, while the poultry population had increased 1,000-fold to 13 billion. Factory farms where large numbers of genetically similar animals are raised and fed in concentrated areas are more common now, especially in the United States and other domesticated countries. Not surprisingly, many emerging infectious diseases have their origin within these animal species.

Long ago, new infectious diseases were spread only as fast and as far as people could walk. Then, use of horses extended the range of contagions. From there, ships sailed on the seas and began to take along germs to whole new worlds. Now, in an age of true global access, the current reach, volume, and speed of travel is unprecedented, and the statistics related to this are impressive:

- Human mobility has increased in high-income countries by over 1,000-fold since 1800.
- Passenger numbers via air travel have grown at nearly 9 percent per year since 1960 and are expected to increase at more than 5 percent per year for at least the next 10 years; airfreight traffic is expected to show similar changes.
- Travel between regions has increased faster than travel within regions.
- There has been a shift in areas visited by travelers, especially to regions in Asia and sub-Saharan Africa.
- Globalization of the world economy has resulted in a shipping traffic increase of over 27 percent since 1993.
- Introduction of risky trade practices that move plants, animals, and other materials (especially in food production and medicine) has influenced microbial spread.

In the setting of increasing human and animal population, our ongoing history of armed conflict has also influenced global spread of disease. Wartime contributes to increased incidence of infectious diseases due to a number of consequences:

- Promotion of violence and war-related injuries: The medical needs of fallen war personnel strain resources and staff, while the injuries themselves can increase an individual's risk of infection.
- Reduced availability of medical care and public health services: Doctors, nurses, and other health care workers are injured or killed (or they flee); clinics and hospitals may be damaged, while supplies of medications and vaccines are reduced, and public health services are stalled.
- Damage to the environment: Food supplies can be contaminated, water safety can be compromised while stagnant water can fill bomb

craters, electrical power can be shut down, and transportation and communication may be interrupted.

- Forced migration of people: As of 2010, there were approximately 12 million refugees and 22–25 million internally displaced persons suffering from loss of sociocultural support systems and reduced access to safe food and water.
- Violations of human rights: Mass abduction of children and rape as a weapon can increase vulnerability to sexually transmitted diseases.
- Diversion of resources: Financing war diverts money from health care to military expenses.
- Use of biological weapons: Examples throughout history have included contaminating drinking water with microorganisms, hurling of plague victims into walled cities, infecting blankets with smallpox, disposing of dead animals in water sources, infecting horses with bacteria, and testing anthrax bombs on a deserted island.

Thus, the impressive global growth of economic activity, tourism, trade, wars, and human migration has resulted in the increased movement of infectious agents and their disease vectors. Perhaps not surprisingly, influenza was the primary infectious disease that was clearly influenced by the growing global transportation in the twentieth century; it was also the principal infectious agent to display pandemic behavior in that same timeline. We are now able to reach almost any destination across the globe within the incubation period for most pathogens, including influenza. In addition, travel for humans is discontinuous (there are many stops and layovers along the way); this influences the movement of pathogens as well. As travel has shifted to low-latitude countries, humans are exposed to areas that have greater species richness, but often poor sanitation and limited infrastructure, which can facilitate spread of disease.

Remember that the flu is often spread via respiratory droplets expelled into the environment by the cough or sneeze of an infected person and that these droplets can reach people up to six feet away. This means that the flu can spread very easily from person to person in areas of close contact, such as airplanes and trains. As an individual traveler, there are steps you can take to protect yourself and others from influenza:

- First and foremost, get the flu vaccine before you travel and be sure to return for vaccination every year.
- Don't travel if you are ill.
- Prepare a travel health kit, including tissues, pain and/or fever medications, soap, hand sanitizer, and sanitizing wipes.
- Wash your hands frequently throughout your travels. If you don't have ready access to water, use hand sanitizer.

- Cover your mouth and nose with a tissue when you cough or sneeze. If you don't have a tissue handy, use your upper arm.
- Don't touch your eyes, nose, or mouth. If you find yourself touching your face, stop and then go wash your hands with soap and water or use hand sanitizer.
- Wash your hands after touching shared spaces such as door handles, seat buckles, and seats on transportation.
- Use your sanitary wipes to clean the armrests, tray tables, and seatbelts when you board your flight or train. If you are staying in a hotel, use the wipes to disinfect the television remote, the toilet handle, elevator buttons, and other frequently touched surfaces.
- Stay away from people who are coughing and sneezing (remain more than six feet apart if possible).
- Drink plenty of water, which helps keep your temperature normal and helps get rid of waste. Avoid too many caffeinated beverages.

Of note, numerous approaches have been developed to predict the possible future movements of infectious agents such as influenza through both local and global transportation networks. When it comes to epidemics, the growth and movement is related primarily to the number of sick people that arises from an initial ill person within an entirely susceptible population and the average time it takes for those secondary cases to become infected. Pandemics, by definition, are much more unpredictable than epidemics, but the study of previous pandemics is necessary so that attempts at both prevention and control can be undertaken. Pandemic preparation will be discussed further in chapter 10.

THE ANTI-VACCINATION MOVEMENT

As has already been made clear in earlier chapters of this book, vaccines are a major tool for achieving public health success in infectious disease prevention or even eradication. It has also been shown that vaccines are overwhelmingly safe to administer. Yet, for some people, the scientific basis on which vaccines are based, the extensive testing that has proven both efficacy and safety of vaccines, and the opinion of medical providers who recommend adherence to vaccine schedules is not enough to convince them to proceed with vaccination; this attitude is known as vaccine hesitancy. Unfortunately, vaccine hesitancy can lead to outright refusal of vaccination, and unvaccinated clusters of humans allow for emergence of the diseases the vaccines were intended to prevent. The World Health

Organization (WHO) has identified vaccine hesitancy as one of the top 10 global health threats of 2019.

As you might remember from chapter 2, the process of variolation met with resistance as attempts to reduce the disease and deaths due to smallpox were made in the eighteenth century; thus, anti-immunization philosophies actually preceded the development of vaccines. Though a lot of the early opposition to vaccines was theological (vaccines were thought to be the devil's work or an attempt to oppose God's punishments upon man for his sins), there were also political and legal objections. In Britain, passage of laws made it mandatory for parents to vaccinate their children in the mid-nineteenth century. This was followed by the formation of the Anti-Vaccination League in London with a clear mission: to protect the liberties of the people who were considered compromised by the mandated vaccine laws. Opposition to vaccines has continued into contemporary times, and the anti-vaccination movement has achieved a particular prominence now. Researchers have documented a clear increase in parental concerns about vaccines; in a survey conducted in 2000, only 19 percent of parents expressed concerns about vaccinations, while in 2009, this jumped to 50 percent. By 2011, another study suggested that 77 percent of parents had concerns about one or more childhood vaccinations.

The current anti-vaccination movement can be traced to the 1980–1990s. In 1982, a television documentary aired on the subject of a proposed link between the pertussis vaccine and seizures in young children. Doctors criticized the show for its inaccuracies, but the fear of vaccines started anew. Then, in 1998, a former British physician named Andrew Wakefield published a paper in *The Lancet*, a well-known and well-respected medical journal. The paper reported a study of 12 children who were diagnosed with autism; Wakefield suggested that the diagnosis of autism in these children was linked to the measles-mumps-rubella (MMR) vaccine. It was later found that Wakefield had been paid by a lawyer through the UK Legal Aid Fund to conduct "scientific research" and provide "expert testimony" that would be featured in litigation on behalf of 1600 families claiming that the MMR vaccine did harm. Further investigation into Wakefield's study also found that clinicians and pathology services at the hospital where Wakefield worked had found nothing to implicate the MMR vaccine. Clinical records of the study were found to differ with the results in the published paper, and changes in the diagnoses, histories, and descriptions of the 12 children were discovered. It even came to light that Wakefield had paid kids at his son's birthday party for their blood samples. Further, in a press conference, Wakefield stated that giving children an MMR vaccine in three separate single doses would be safer than one combined vaccine; it was later found that Wakefield had already applied for a patent for a new single vaccine before participating in the press conference.

Investigations led to retraction of Wakefield's paper by *The Lancet* in 2010, and Wakefield was found to have acted dishonestly and irresponsibly; his medical license in the United Kingdom was taken away. He ultimately left England and moved to America. Subsequent peer-reviewed studies have not shown any association between the MMR vaccine and autism. However, the damage was already done—the anti-vaccination movement was kick-started, and Wakefield achieved the status of martyr among anti-vaccination believers. Wakefield's false statements about the MMR vaccine had global repercussions as they spread from the United Kingdom to Western Europe and North America. In the four years between 1996 and 2002, MMR vaccination rates in the United Kingdom dropped from 92 percent to 84 percent and even reached 61 percent in some parts of London in 2003. In Ireland, the national immunization level fell below 80 percent by 1999–2000. In the United States, MMR vaccine rates declined by 2 percent in 1999–2000. These declines resulted in multiple breakouts of measles throughout the Western world. Indeed, Wakefield's fraudulent findings have been identified as the most damaging medical hoax in 100 years.

It is easy to think that people might have vaccine hesitancy because they suffer from a deficit of information about vaccines, they lack access to the facts, or they are misinformed by people such as Wakefield as to the success and safety of vaccines. Known as the information deficit model of science communication, this suggests that providing additional factual information will fill the knowledge gap and help move people toward vaccination. However, this clearly doesn't explain the current anti-vaccination movement. Indeed, information alone has not been shown to increase vaccine confidence among hesitant parents. The now-global reach of the anti-vaccination movement has resulted in pockets of vaccine refusal that exist in many communities; these areas with low vaccination rates have resulted in localized outbreaks of vaccine-preventable disease like measles and pertussis. Believe it or not, the arguments against vaccination have actually changed little over time, though they are continually updated to better reflect more modern science, contemporary language, and advancements in technology. A variety of influential individuals and organizations circulate the anti-vaccination arguments that are then read and repeated by parents and other media consumers. In addition to the information concerns, the three biggest reasons for vaccine hesitancy fall into these categories: (a) safety concerns, (b) personal beliefs and philosophical reasons, and (c) religious reasons. Religious reasons are generally the reflection of the core beliefs of parents and most often result in a complete refusal of *all* vaccinations. Some of the most often expressed issues within the categories of vaccine safety and/or personal beliefs about vaccination are listed here:

MYTH: *Vaccines are toxic because they contain dangerous chemicals or substances such as thimerosal (mercury), formaldehyde, aluminum, antifreeze, and aborted fetal tissues.*
FACT: Thimerosal is an antifungal agent used to preserve multi-dose vials of vaccine in order to vaccinate many people from one vial. Thimerosal has a mercury atom in it; this ethyl mercury gets flushed out of the body, unlike methyl mercury (like that found in tuna). In an effort to appease the anti-vaccination crowd, thimerosal was removed from vaccines for children under six years of age in 2000, even though there had been no link between it and autism. Now, people in developing nations have to pay more money to buy and maintain single-dose vials of vaccines because the preserved multi-dose vials are no longer available. With regard to the other substances, formaldehyde is naturally found in plants, animals, and humans. The level of formaldehyde found in your body is 100 times greater than that which is found in a vaccine. Aluminum is present in low levels in vaccines in order to produce a better immune response; the amount of aluminum in a vaccine is 1/100th of our daily consumption, and it has never been shown to be harmful. Antifreeze and aborted fetal tissues have never been used in vaccines.

MYTH: *Vaccines aren't actually effective in preventing infectious diseases.*
FACT: One common misperception among those who express vaccine hesitancy is that vaccines aren't actually effective. The opposite is true, and to put it simply, vaccines might actually be a victim of their own success. As a disease becomes less common or even eradicated after widespread vaccination, common knowledge about that infection is decreased in the general population, and recognition of the potentially dangerous (or fatal) consequences of that infection is even less known. In turn, it can be more challenging for public health institutions and health care providers to articulate the desirability of vaccination against a disease for which people have only a vague appreciation. Some studies on vaccine behaviors have delineated the difference between "active demand" (getting vaccinated due to an appreciation of the benefits of and the need for vaccination) and "passive acceptance" (undergoing vaccination in compliance with recommendations from an authority). Demand, which might more easily influence people to overcome their vaccine hesitancy, is often low in our contemporary times because we don't remember the terrible symptoms and risk of death associated with diseases such as polio and measles. Ensuring compliance and high coverage rates via

passive acceptance becomes even more difficult as the anti-vaccination movement spreads.

MYTH: *Most of the infections that vaccines attempt to prevent aren't dangerous anyway.*
FACT: Some of the world's worst infectious diseases in history are less known to us today because they have been controlled or eradicated due to vaccination. To think that infection with these pathogens would be rare or that these pathogens would be of minimal consequence even without vaccines is both irresponsible and incorrect. In a recent large-scale review on vaccine behavior, perceiving a lack of benefit to the vaccine and perceiving oneself as less susceptible to the disease were both barriers to receiving the influenza vaccine. Vaccination rates were also less in individuals who had not suffered from influenza previously. Yet, as you might recall from the introduction to this book, influenza infects between 5 and 15 percent of the world's population *each year,* with even higher numbers in children (about 30 percent). A more recent study looking at seasonal flu between 2010 and 2018 in the United States has shown that the virus resulted in up to 23 million medical visits, almost a million hospitalizations, and up to 79,000 respiratory and circulatory deaths *each year.* Worldwide, it has been estimated that up to 645,000 respiratory deaths are associated with influenza annually.

MYTH: *It is better to have natural immunity from being exposed to the infectious disease itself than it is to achieve artificial immunity through vaccination.*
FACT: While natural immunity from catching a disease can occasionally offer stronger immunity to the disease than a vaccination, the dangers of the disease far outweigh the benefits. The risk of having a serious adverse reaction to a vaccine is one in a million. But the risk of complications from an infection that vaccines could have prevented is closer to 1 in 100 to 1 in 1,000. In addition, some vaccines (such as those targeting genital warts, a bacterium named *Haemophilus,* and tetanus) provide better immunity than the disease itself.

MYTH: *A child's immune system can become overloaded by the vaccination schedule.*
FACT: Based on the number of antibodies present in the blood, babies would theoretically have the ability to respond to around 10,000 vaccines at once. The small number of compounds found in vaccines is far less than the number of compounds produced by the thousands of germs that babies are exposed to every day. And even though there are more vaccines than ever before, they are much more efficient—small children are

actually exposed to fewer immunological components than kids in past decades.

MYTH: *Vaccines can actually cause the disease they are trying to prevent (e.g., the influenza vaccine causes the flu).*
FACT: While vaccines can cause mild symptoms resembling those of the disease they are protecting against, these symptoms *are not due to infection.* Rather, the symptoms are the result of activation of the body's immune system, which is exactly the response you'd want from a vaccine that is attempting to trigger immune system protection. As you might remember from the discussion of vaccines in chapter 8, the IIVs, ccIIV, and RIV all contain inactivated influenza viral strains and thus *cannot* cause the flu. LAIVs contain attenuated live influenza viral strains and thus *cannot* cause the flu.

MYTH: *There is no need to get vaccinated personally if other people are already vaccinated and there is low risk of transmitting the disease to others, anyway.*
FACT: Herd immunity is the key to limiting the ability of an infectious disease to establish itself and spread onward in a community, and it is absolutely necessary given that there will always be a part of the population that cannot be vaccinated or are at high risk for complications of infection (infants, the elderly, pregnant women, and immunocompromised people, to name a few). However, there is a level of vaccination a population must achieve to allow for herd immunity to be effective. This vaccination threshold is variable depending on how contagious an infectious agent might be. For polio, the minimum percentage of immune individuals needed to establish herd immunity is 80–86 percent. The vaccine threshold increases to 93–95 percent for measles, which is so contagious that a single person can infect up to 90 percent of the people around them if they are not immune. For influenza, the threshold is estimated to be about 80 percent.

Other specific reasons cited by individuals for their vaccine hesitancy have included distrust of pharmaceutical companies; belief in alternative medicine; a feeling that choices of vaccines are too limited (or alternatively, that there are too many vaccine choices); fear of needles; a feeling that one is too old for vaccination; lack of access to vaccines due to political, geographical, or economic issues; distrust of government sources; and lack of time to get vaccinated. Studies have even shown that there are certain physical barriers that are associated with reduced influenza vaccination, including alcohol consumption, tobacco use (interestingly, though, having given up smoking was noted to increase the likelihood of vaccination), level of physical activity (mixed results with low level of physical activity reported as a barrier to vaccination for some but perceived "good" health status resulting in less inclination for vaccination in others), lower body mass index, and no preexisting medical conditions. In a recent review of vaccine behavior studies over a 10-year period, 29 separate studies identified "social benefit" as an influence on influenza vaccination. Social benefit (meaning "it's the right thing to do") is not an uncommon argument in favor of vaccination. Sadly, those who do not acknowledge the social benefit of the influenza vaccine are less likely to be vaccinated, including health care providers who lack the belief that getting vaccinated protects patients and pregnant women who lack the belief that the vaccine would offer benefit to their unborn child. Individuals who perceive that there is low risk in transmitting the flu to others also have decreased vaccination rates.

Not unexpectedly, the internet is used frequently as a source of vaccination information, for both good and bad. It has been demonstrated that 80 percent of individuals use the internet yearly to search for health information, but relatively few discuss these findings with a medical professional. Celebrity anti-vaccination influencers are particularly effective at spreading misinformation online via social media. Perhaps the biggest name associated with the contemporary anti-vaccination movement is Jenny McCarthy, an actress and comedian who is the parent of an autistic child. She has over a million followers on Facebook alone and has authored several books that have promoted an anti-vaccine philosophy. Other women known as "Mommy Bloggers" have also been influential in reaching people online, including the following:

- Sarah Pope: Nutrition and parenting blogger who is known as the "Healthy Home Economist"
- Megan Redshaw: Mother and "wellness" blogger who posts self-declared "common sense" information, including avoidance of vaccines
- Kate Tietje: Mother of five who blogs at "Modern Alternative Momma" and sells "health and wellness" products online
- Vani Hari: Influential "food safety" blogger who recommends against vaccines

An analysis of anti-vaccination websites has demonstrated that the great majority of sites (every website examined except one) "contained arguments against vaccination that could be considered disingenuous." The "Mommy Blogs" were also analyzed and found to tell persuasive stories suggesting that vaccines pose a threat to children. A study that examined the content of the first 100 sites found after searching for "vaccination" and "immunization" on Google concluded that 43 percent of the websites were anti-vaccination, including all of the first 10.

Another significant contributor to vaccine hesitancy appears to be erosion of public trust in institutions involved with vaccination. With the general public more enamored with ideas of individual empowerment and patient choice, public health entities that issue vaccine recommendations have less and less influence. Yet, anti-vaccination online organizers have been successful in adding to vaccine hesitancy, including the following:

- J. B. Handley: Activist and parent of an autistic child who cofounded two organizations that suggest vaccines are a major factor driving development of autism
- Robert F. Kennedy Jr.: Environmental lawyer who authored both a book (*Thimerosal: Let the Science Speak*) and an article ("Deadly Immunity"), which was ultimately retracted from *Rolling Stone* and *Salon*
- Barbara Loe Fisher: Activist, author, and founder of the National Vaccine Information Center who began speaking out against vaccines after her son suffered what she believes to be a vaccine injury
- Mike Adams: Owner/operator of "Natural News" and purveyor of conspiracy theories, suggesting the government is lying to the public about vaccines and other infectious issues

Health care providers often become vaccinated because of their personal belief in the benefits of vaccine, as well as out of a sense of duty to their patients and their communities. Unfortunately, this doesn't hold true for all health care professionals. Indeed, some individual anti-vaccine influencers, such as Andrew Wakefield, are doctors, including the following:

- Robert Sears: California physician and author of *The Vaccine Book*, which formulated an "alternative" vaccine schedule that delays many vaccines from the CDC-recommended guidelines
- Sherri Tenpenny: Private practice physician in Ohio and author of several books that argue against vaccination and cofounder of the International Medical Council on Vaccination, whose purpose is to "counter the messages asserted by pharmaceutical companies, the government, and medical agencies that vaccines are safe, effective, and harmless"
- Toni Bark: Now deceased; previously a private practice physician at the Center for Disease Prevention and Reversal
- Susanne Humphries: Private practice physician in Maine and Virginia and author of *Dissolving Illusions: Disease, Vaccines, and the Forgotten History*

- Larry Palevsky: Private practice physician and holistic/integrative physician in New York
- Joseph Mercola: Former private practice physician in Illinois who now runs the business Mercola.com and author of *The Great Bird Flu Hoax: The Truth They Don't Want You to Know about the "Next Big Pandemic"*

A recent review of studies on influenza vaccination behaviors noted that health care personnel who lacked the belief that the vaccine was an ethical or professional obligation were less likely to be vaccinated; they also were less often vaccinated for the flu if they did not acknowledge that it was their duty to do no harm and to ensure continuity of care. However, achieving herd immunity is clearly in the best interest of society as a whole, and health care providers should feel they are able to offer vaccinations and vaccine information to their patients without ethical repercussions. Certainly, better education for health care providers regarding vaccines may help clarify their own personal beliefs; it has been shown that a lack of influenza-specific education results in decreased vaccination among health care providers. Another way to promote health care provider self-vaccination is to remove any practical barriers to workplace vaccination, to offer free vaccinations, and to recognize that vaccination helps providers avoid absenteeism.

It has been shown that a trustful doctor-patient relationship is absolutely necessary for providers to successfully recommend vaccines to patients. A recent large-scale review of vaccine behaviors showed that individuals who did not receive a direct recommendation from medical personnel were frequently reported to be less likely to vaccinate. It is crucial, then, that providers feel they can safely and effectively have this conversation with their patients. There are at least three challenges reported by health care professionals when it comes to building a trustful relationship with their patients. Firstly, providers feel they don't have enough time with their patients to engage in a thoughtful complete conversation about vaccination.

Secondly, some health care providers suffer from a lack of awareness about vaccination guidelines and/or have a lack of adequate knowledge about vaccines in general. And even if the provider is informed, they may not feel confident in sharing their expertise. In one dataset review of vaccination beliefs, providers could be categorized based on whether they were assertive or unassertive. Unassertive providers were easily perturbed by their environment (such as a media scare) with regard to their vaccine beliefs, while assertive providers carried a stable belief in the value of vaccination. In addition to some of the myths already discussed previously, some health care providers have expressed the following false beliefs: (a) pregnancy is a contraindication for the pandemic influenza vaccine, (b) vaccines promote allergies, and (c) seasonal influenza vaccine also protects against pandemic influenza. Health care providers need to have accurate information about the efficacy and safety of vaccines and to feel that they can be assertive in their communication with patients. Thirdly, some health care providers support vaccination as a general preventative measure, but they have some personal reservations about specific vaccines (this has been a particular problem with the vaccination for human papilloma virus, which is a sexually transmitted pathogen).

So, what can be done to combat the anti-vaccination movement? Clearly, this is an exceedingly complicated and difficult societal health threat that has global consequences.

- Though it is clear that information alone cannot perfectly deter vaccine hesitancy, providing reliable facts to those who genuinely seek science-based evidence about vaccination remains essential. For the general public, such information can be provided to friends or family members, submitted to local newspapers as opinion pieces or letters to editors, or provided online via blog posts, social media updates, or on other internet sites.
- State legislators should be contacted to advocate for the strengthening of vaccine exemption policies. Although there are no federal laws regarding vaccine administration, each state has laws in place dictating whether or not children must be vaccinated prior to entering schools. Unfortunately, many states allow exemption from vaccination for medical, religious, and/or philosophical reasons. It has been proven that states with stricter exemption criteria have higher rates of vaccine compliance. Though anti-vaccination proponents might argue that this is an infringement upon autonomy, public health policymakers should understand that state-regulated vaccinations for all children is justified using rule utilitarianism (the ideology that a rule for society should be established that has the best outcome for the greatest number of people in the society).
- If a state has a religious exemption policy in place, there should be requirements that mandate parents to demonstrate genuine and sincere beliefs (essentially, a burden of proof) that contradict the use of vaccines.
- We need to restore trust and credibility in institutions involved in vaccination.
- Improvement is needed in the design of teaching curricula and training programs of health care professionals with regard to vaccines, the myths surrounding vaccinations, and the skills needed to engage

patients in conversations about vaccinations, especially if vaccine hesitancy is identified.

- Support should be given to health care professionals, as they are the main and most influential source of vaccination information and they are instrumental in helping their patients move past vaccine hesitancy toward vaccine compliance.
- Physician offices could create "vaccine ambassador" programs to accommodate parents who are interested in speaking out and promoting vaccination.
- As a society, we need to hold firm to the idea that vaccination is "normal" and expected, especially when considering that a parent's motivation to vaccinate their children is influenced by social norms.
- We need to help shape online and social media influence, including stories of uncomplicated vaccine administrations that occur every day without incident.
- There should be improved systems for post-vaccination monitoring, which can provide an avenue for conversation about concerns for adverse reactions and post-vaccination anxieties.

10

Current Research and Future Directions

As the previous chapters have already made clear, influenza will likely continue to cause seasonal outbreaks for years to come. Unfortunately, most scientists also agree that another influenza pandemic is only a matter of time. What, then, can ongoing research add to what we already know about the virus, its prevention, and the methods of treatment? And can we ever learn enough to mitigate a global catastrophe should another pandemic occur?

RESEARCH ON TREATMENT AND PREVENTION

While we already know a lot about the influenza virus and methods of both prevention (vaccination and chemoprophylaxis) and treatment (antiviral medications and supportive care) exist, there is still much to accomplish with ongoing research and development.

Treatment

Though much attention has focused on vaccine development in order to prevent infection with influenza, there will always be people who can't receive the flu vaccine or in whom the vaccination may not offer perfect protection. Thus, researchers around the globe are trying to develop more antiviral medications that might help in treating influenza infection should it occur. One scientist in the United States is conducting research that focuses on the mutation in the M2 channel. You might remember from chapter 5 that a mutation in the M2 channel has resulted in resistance of the influenza virus to the antiviral class of M2 inhibitors, which includes amantadine and rimantadine. If the mutation can be reversed or inhibited in some way, then we could use these antiviral medications that are already available for treatment of the flu, saving time and money in terms of drug production and release to the public. Other ongoing research projects are focused on the influenza virus's polymerase. The antiviral class of endonuclease inhibitors use this approach as well, but with a different target on the HA protein. One new antiviral drug under development in this class, named pimodivir, inhibits a specific aspect of the polymerase complex. One clinical trial using pimodivir has included hospitalized patients, while another clinical trial involves outpatients who are at high risk of complications from influenza.

In addition to the research that focuses on development of new antiviral medications, another investigation is underway to find known compounds that might be effective as treatment or adjuncts ("boosters" that can improve the success of other antiviral treatments) for influenza. Uricosuric agents, a class of medications that inhibit the kidney secretion of the active metabolite of oseltamivir, are one category of medications that has already been proposed for adjunct use. Probenecid, an existing drug in the uricosuric category, has been found to reduce the clearance of oseltamivir by approximately 50 percent while doubling the body's exposure to the antiviral medicine. Though use of probenecid as an adjunctive therapy with oseltamivir in the treatment of avian influenza has been proposed, appropriate dosing has not yet been established; hopefully, more concrete recommendations for use of this adjunct will be forthcoming with further research. Other researchers in France have identified 31 previously FDA-approved molecules that show promising antiviral activity. Of those 31 molecules, one calcium-channel-blocker (a medicine normally used to treat high blood pressure) has demonstrated potential benefit against the influenza virus when tested in mice. A clinical trial to test its ability to offer treatment for humans infected with the flu is underway.

Other investigators are considering the use of antibodies to fight the influenza virus. You may remember that antibodies are produced by our immune system to target and defeat infectious agents like viruses. As was described in chapter 1, binding of the HA on the flu virus to the sialic acid receptors on our respiratory tract epithelial cells allows entry of the virus into the cell. A group of investigators in the United Kingdom have attached extra sialic acids to part of an antibody. In theory, when the virus encounters these antibodies, it would bind to the sialic-acid-coated antibodies *instead* of the sialic acid found on the surface of host lung cells. This would prevent viral invasion into the cells, which prohibits further viral replication and halts the infectious process.

Prevention

Though there are lots of ways we try to limit our risks for becoming ill, the primary measure of prevention against influenza is, of course, vaccination. However, as was mentioned in chapter 8, there are a lot of issues involving the selection, manufacturing, and production of influenza vaccines, including the following.

Variable Degrees of Efficacy

To date, the vaccines against influenza have been relatively weak in their ability to stimulate a vigorous immune response (immunogenicity). In addition, there is also waning immunity that comes with age, known as immunosenescence; this means the elderly have particularly poor responsiveness to vaccines. Thus, ongoing research is needed to improve the immune system's response to the flu vaccine, especially in at-risk target populations like the elderly.

One way to improve immunogenicity is with the use of vaccine adjuvants, which are compounds that can enhance the immune response elicited by an antigen. Some of these adjuvants include aluminum salt (alum) and the squalene oil-in-water emulsion systems called MF59 and AS03. Although alum has been used successfully in other vaccines, the benefit in influenza H5N1 vaccines has been limited so far; however, the MF59 adjuvant has been more promising. Adjuvanted vaccines induce a stronger immune response in the elderly (>65 years of age) and have double the efficacy of unadjuvanted formulations in young children, too—these are two of the high-risk populations of concern. Other newer adjuvants that are being tested are immunostimulatory DNA sequences and bacterium-derived components, which are both expected to enhance the innate and adaptive immune responses. Another approach to increasing the immunogenicity of the influenza vaccine is via alternative delivery routes. Research of further intradermal inoculations and other types of delivery systems is ongoing.

Variable Viruses

In order for a vaccine to be most effective, there must be a good match between the strains of virus included in the vaccine and the strains that circulate in the community during seasonal flu. Current strategies to address this mismatch include improvement of global surveillance and-development of new-generation vaccines that target regions of the virus that don't mutate from year to year.

In the second half of the 2018–2019 influenza season, it was discovered that a drifted H3N2 variant had emerged. Studies found that the influenza vaccine for that season was not protective against this variant strain. This finding prompted WHO to postpone choosing an H3N2 virus for the northern hemisphere's 2019–2020 influenza vaccine, which then ultimately delayed vaccine shipments in the United States. (This type of delay was not unprecedented; this was the third time since 2000 that a vaccine strain selection was postponed so that additional data could be collected to help choose the best-matched strain.) In analyzing data from the Flu Vaccine Effectiveness Network, it was found that while H1N1 viruses were prominent in the first half of the influenza season, the variant H3N2 viruses predominated in the second half, contributing to the longest influenza season in the United States in 10 years. The vaccine was estimated to be 44 percent effective against the H1N1 strains but only 9 percent effective against H3N2 strains overall. Thus, some scientists have proposed that creating a pentavalent vaccine (one containing five different viral strains) is worthy of discussion; this would allow a second H3N2 strain to be added to the mix. Since it was initially proposed, this idea has since been suggested to be unrealistic due to an inability to predict emergence of drifted strains in the middle of the influenza season and the limitations of our current vaccine production models.

Limited Vaccine Availability

There are great differences in vaccine availability in countries throughout the world. Cheaper vaccines that induce longer-lasting immunity are needed, as are better vaccine distribution avenues across the globe.

Limitations in Manufacturing and Production Time

The optimal period of time between selection of the viral strains for the vaccine and delivery of the vaccine is short, and there is little room for unanticipated delays, as has already been noted. The requirement for larger quantities of vaccine as populations grow also imposes a production burden on the manufacturing process. In order to combat these limitations, strategies are needed to improve the growth of conventional vaccine viruses, reduce the production time, and improve manufacturing processes.

Egg-based vaccine production has served its purpose for many years, but it is an intensive process that requires too many resources and too much time. It is also dependent upon a continuous supply of eggs; concerns about contamination of the egg supply by avian pathogens, contamination of the eggs with microbials during processing, and limited egg supply during a pandemic, as well as risk of adverse effects in people with egg allergies, have prompted consideration of alternative strategies for inoculation of viral cultures. One of these newer strategies was mentioned in chapter 8: the use of cell culture platforms. Growth of influenza in a cell culture platform has advantages in terms of scalability, availability, and ease of manipulation; it also negates the egg allergy concerns (eliminating a reason for vaccine hesitancy in some people) and results in fewer adaptive mutations in the growing influenza viruses. One cell culture–based inactivated influenza vaccine was made available during the 2019–2020 influenza season; further work with this production model continues. Other new technologies that are under investigation in the manufacturing of influenza vaccines include the following:

- Implementation of reverse genetics, which utilizes molecular techniques to generate a specific viral strain.
- Use of the baculovirus expression vector system (DNA viruses that produce a specific protein that can be used as a production vehicle). This process was used in the development of the recombinant influenza vaccine that was available for the 2019–2020 flu season.
- Utilization of virus-like particles that have no genetic component, but still retain the morphology and antigenicity of the whole virus.
- Development of viral vector systems using other viruses, such as adenovirus, poxvirus, parainfluenza virus, and alphavirus, which are designed to allow direct delivery to the mucosal site in order to mimic the process of natural influenza virus infection without the presence of the actual flu virus.
- Revisiting DNA vaccines (although this is not exactly a new technology, DNA vaccines have the theoretical benefits of rapid production and ease of immunogen exchange).

Lack of Lifelong Immunity

As you likely remember, influenza vaccines are unable to produce long-lasting antibody titers due to ongoing viral mutations, which is why we have to get vaccinated each year for influenza. In 2008, as was noted in chapter 2, researchers discovered a specific human antibody that protects against a broad spectrum of influenza viruses. With this discovery came the realization that humans were capable of producing antibodies against a part of the influenza virus that doesn't change because of mutation from season to season. If a vaccine could be developed that allows for this particular antibody to be produced, then vaccination against influenza might offer lifelong immunity. A universal influenza vaccine would be an extraordinary medical achievement.

One target that is being explored for the universal vaccine is the extracellular domain of the M2 protein, known as M2e. Although the exact mechanism of M2e-specific immunity is not entirely clear, research on mice has shown that vaccination with a baculovirus-derived M2 protected them from death from the H1N1 and H3N2 viral strains. Another target for a universal influenza vaccine has been cytotoxic T lymphocytes (CTLs), which are a component of the human immune response. There have been several research projects using different approaches to increase the numbers of CTLs through vaccination. In humans who have not yet produced an antibody to a specific influenza strain, a robust CTL response is crucial for early clearance of the virus; CTL vaccines would provide baseline immunity in this population with the hope of protection against a newly emerging pandemic virus in the future. Another universal influenza vaccine concept in development involves cross-reactive HA stalk antibodies. It has long been known that cross-reactive antibodies that target the HA stalk can be induced, but they are produced in only small amounts after infection. If the HA stalk antibodies can be induced at protective levels, this could potentially result in long-lasting immunity.

CONCERNS FOR A FUTURE PANDEMIC

As noted in chapter 1, a pandemic is a large-scale epidemic of an infectious disease causing extraordinary morbidity and mortality over a wide geographic (global) area, resulting in significant economic, social, and political disruption. In general, pandemics appear to be increasing in frequency, likely because of the increasing emergence of viral strains originating from animals. When asked if there is a risk of a future influenza pandemic, most science experts answer unequivocally: *yes*. Despite the medical advances we've made in the last century, the likelihood of pandemics has actually increased because of greater human and avian/swine populations, global travel and integration, changes in land use, more exploitation of the natural environment, and the anti-vaccination movement.

Unfortunately, when compared to other pathogens, influenza is one of the infectious agents most likely to cause a severe pandemic. It has been estimated that in any given year, a 1 percent probability exists of an influenza pandemic that could cause nearly 6 million pneumonia- and flu-related deaths across the globe. An influenza pandemic having a global death rate similar to the 2009 Swine flu pandemic has about a 3 percent probability of occurrence in any given year. Why is influenza more likely to cause a severe pandemic than other pathogens? It is the principal threat because of a number of factors:

- Influenza has a high rate of mutation (antigenic shift and drift) with inclusion of genetic material from animal (swine and avian) sources.
- Strains of the influenza virus continue to be in seasonal rotation year after year.
- Human-to-human transmission of many influenza strains is efficient and successful.
- The incubation period of influenza is long enough to allow undetected movement of infected but asymptomatic individuals.
- The symptomatic profile of influenza causes difficulty in diagnosis (symptoms of the flu mimic other respiratory infections that are less worrisome, such as the common cold).

Some literature has suggested that the likelihood of a pandemic is driven by two factors: spark risk and spread risk. Spark risk is *where* a pandemic is likely to arise, while spread risk is *how likely* it is to diffuse broadly through the human population. One spark risk for influenza is obviously zoonotic: the introduction of a pathogen from domesticated animals (such as swine or poultry) or wildlife (such as waterfowl) that can cause disease in humans. Domesticated animals result in increased spark risk due to factory farming and livestock production systems, live markets, and contact between livestock and wildlife reservoirs. Other behavioral factors can contribute to influenza's zoonotic spark risk, such as use of animal-based traditional medicines, natural resource extraction like logging, extension of roads into wildlife habitats, and degree and distribution of animal diversity. Spread risk for influenza is influenced by viral-specific factors (such as genetic mutations and efficacy of transmission) and human population factors (such as density of the population, immunity status, patterns of movement, and speed and success of public health measures).

In 2019, the Global Preparedness Monitoring Board (an independent monitoring and advocacy body known as GPMB) published an annual report on global preparedness for health emergencies. According to this report, between 2011 and 2018, WHO traced 1483 epidemic events in 172 countries. They stated, without hesitation, that virulent respiratory pathogens like influenza pose particular risks for a global emergency such as a pandemic for a number of reasons: they are spread via respiratory droplets, they can infect a large number of people very quickly, and they can move rapidly across multiple geographies in today's transportation infrastructure. The GPMB also clearly stated that the world is *not* prepared for a fast-moving pandemic. Some of the identified preparedness problems that were cited in the report include

- insufficient national and local leadership, as well as inadequate international support, for preparedness in the poorest countries;
- poor integration between preparedness and day-to-day health needs with grossly insufficient involvement of communities in all aspects of preparedness, especially with regard to inclusion of women and youth;
- lack of data sharing and medical countermeasures in the context of a Public Health Emergency of International Concern;
- broken national financing systems for preparedness with insufficient rapid financing and rapid response surge capacity;
- insufficient financing to the poorest countries and ineffective utilization of available funds;
- underfunding of WHO;
- unfit international coordination mechanisms for health emergencies in complex environments; and
- unclear leadership roles should a global event occur.

Based on these inadequacies, the GPMB called for seven urgent actions to prepare the world for possible global health emergencies such as an influenza pandemic:

- Heads of government must commit to preparedness and invest in preparedness as an integral part of national and global security.
- Countries and regional organizations must lead by example and follow through on their political and funding commitments for preparedness.
- All countries much build strong systems for preparedness.
- Countries, donors, and multilateral institutions much be prepared for the worst, such as a rapidly spreading pandemic due to a lethal respiratory pathogen like influenza.
- Financing institutions must link preparedness with financial risk planning to mitigate the severe economic impacts of a regional epidemic and/or a global pandemic.
- Development assistance funders must create incentives and increase funding for preparedness.
- The United Nations much strengthen coordination mechanisms.

Lessons from the Past

It is hard to forget the details of the Spanish flu pandemic of 1918 as previously discussed in chapter 2. An estimated 50 million people died through the three waves of this pandemic, and the historical and socioeconomic consequences were monumental. At the time, many Americans thought that the illness must have been due to a weapon unleashed by the German enemy in the midst of World War I; some even called it "the German plague." Others thought that the pandemic must have been due to poisoned air from use of gas or an effect of the masses of putrefying dead. It was only many years later that the influenza virus was discovered and named as the cause of the pandemic.

Scientists have learned an incredible amount about the flu strain that caused the 1918 pandemic, often using extraordinary measures. One of the most famous researchers is John Hultin (1924–). Originally born in Stockholm, Hultin traveled to Iowa for his graduate studies. While there, he proposed that he might be able to find influenza victims of the pandemic of 1918, who had been buried in the permafrost in Alaska. He theorized that if he could excavate the bodies, he could try to extract the virus from their frozen tissues for further study. His early efforts to do exactly that in Nome and Wales in 1951 were unsuccessful; digs in those areas revealed no permafrost, and all of the corpses were fully deteriorated. Hultin moved on to Brevig Mission, where it was known that 72 of the 80 people living there in 1918 had died of the flu and that their bodies were buried in a mass grave. After four days of digging, Hultin found his first flu victim preserved in the permafrost. She was a little girl thought to be 6–10 years old; further digging eventually uncovered four more bodies. Placing small pieces of frozen lung tissue from each body in sterile containers, Hultin returned to the University of Iowa with his samples, though he admittedly had difficulty keeping the tissue frozen on the trip home. Back in his lab, he ground up the tissue, suspended it in a salt solution, and spun it in a centrifuge to separate the virus from debris. He added an antibiotic solution to try to kill off any bacteria that were present and then began injecting the fluid into hundreds of fertilized chick eggs. Sadly, no viral growth occurred. He then tried making other suspensions and injecting the fluid into the nasal passages of guinea pigs, white mice, and ferrets. None of the animals ever became ill. Eventually, Hultin ran out of lung tissue samples, and he was forced to terminate his work; he never wrote up his results or published a paper on the failed experiment.

Jeffrey Taubenberger (1961–), a dual-trained medical doctor/microbiologist and Chief of Molecular Pathology at the National Institute of Health, was also intrigued by the idea of extracting the 1918 flu virus from preserved tissue samples. Taubenberger remembered that Abraham Lincoln, during his tenure as president of the United States, mandated that every military doctor who examined tissue after a patient's death had to send a specimen to be stored in the repository at the Armed Forces Institute of Pathology. Taubenberger also knew he had access to these specimens and that some of them might have been from soldiers who died of the flu during the 1918 pandemic. Sure enough, in the late 1990's, he found 70 such specimens, along with documentation of clinical histories; he chose six of these to study further. He and his team managed to eventually separate the genetic pieces of the 1918 flu virus from these tissue samples, and after many failed attempts, they were finally successful: using the tissue from a 21-year-old soldier from Camp Jackson in South Carolina who died of influenza in September 1918, they were able to match one viral gene after another for influenza, and the strain causing the 1918 pandemic was identified: H1N1. After Taubenberger's success, Hultin actually returned to Alaska on a solo expedition. In Brevig Mission, he excavated the corpse of a young woman whom he called Lucy. Lucy was likely in her mid-twenties when she died of complications of the flu during the 1918 pandemic, and her lungs were found to be perfectly frozen and filled with blood. Hultin took carefully preserved specimens and shipped them to the Armed Forces Institute of Pathology. Within days, he was informed by Dr. Taubenberger's team that the genetic material from the H1N1 virus had been isolated from Lucy's tissue specimens.

Many scientists have now studied the H1N1 virus extensively, and it is thought that the ancestor of this viral strain infected humans sometime between 1900 and 1915; however, it has been postulated that the virus obtained its HA from avian viruses. It isn't entirely clear why this virus was so deadly, especially for young adults between the ages of 20 and 40. Some researchers have speculated that the following reasons might account for the impressive lethality of the this viral strain: (a) it exhibited higher replication rates and virulence of the HA gene; (b) it had enhanced pathogenicity with activation of HA by the NA gene; (c) it had faster replication in host respiratory epithelial cells; and d) it inhibited the host's interferon response. Ultimately, the unique combination of all of the genes of the H1N1 virus made it particularly dangerous; indeed, no other human influenza virus tested has been as deadly.

In addition to the viral factors that were thought to contribute to the severity of the 1918 pandemic, historians have identified other causes that might have influenced the outcomes of this pandemic:

- World War I: The global spread of the disease was clearly facilitated by the movement of troops.
- Female gender: Some women suffered disproportionally, possibly as a result of pregnancy and the demands of acting as caretakers of others.

- Lack of immunity: With H1N1 thought to be a strain of influenza to which few humans had ever been exposed, they had little innate protection against the virus, and influenza vaccines did not exist in 1918.
- Poor leadership: Complacency, incompetency, and effects of illness likely played a role in the inability of federal, state, and city leaders to react to the pandemic in a timely manner, and no coordinated prepandemic plans were available.
- Secondary bacterial infection: There is a high likelihood that many of the deaths in 1918 resulted from a combined effect of influenza and a subsequent bacterial pneumonia. Medical technology to aid in diagnosis was limited, and countermeasures, such as critical care services, antiviral medications, and antibiotics, hadn't been developed yet.
- Shortages in health care providers: The sick outnumbered the available help, leading to deficiencies in medical care, adequate fluids, food, and supportive measures. Up to 30 percent of physicians in the United States were deployed to military service during the pandemic.
- Underlying disease: Those with other medical problems, such as diabetes or heart disease, were more likely to have suffered fatal consequences in the setting of influenza infection.

Because the influenza virus had not yet been discovered in 1918, there were no specific antiviral medications or preventative vaccines available. The flu could only be fought with symptomatic treatments and improvised remedies. The first official preventative measures implemented in the United States in 1918 were obligatory notification of suspected cases of influenza and the surveillance of special communities such as day schools, boarding schools, and military barracks. As the pandemic spread globally, European officials began to add further measures, including the closure of public meeting places (such as theaters) and the suspension of public meetings. Even long church sermons were no longer allowed, and Sunday instruction was to last no more than five minutes. More and more measures were attempted to stop the spread of the flu, including cleaning of the streets, disinfecting of public spaces, banning crowds outside shops, limiting the number of passengers on public transport, establishing voluntary and/or mandatory quarantines, distributing free soap and clean water, aiding in the removal of human waste, inspecting milk and other food products, forbidding spitting in the streets, collecting corpses at specially assigned points, and abolishing death rituals. Though Spain was an exception, many European countries refrained from reporting news of the spreading infection during the pandemic of 1918. This was done in order to prevent alarm and panic in the general population (especially since they were already reeling from the sufferings inflicted by the World War I).

Denial by officials regarding the spread of the pandemic was noted in both national and international newspapers, while hygiene authorities refused to reveal the numbers of people affected and deaths due to the flu. Newspapers were key in spreading word about the public emergency measures to contain the pandemic, while at the same time attempting to limit any mention of the severity of it.

While fascinating to revisit, it is also incredibly important for us to remember these viral factors, historical influences, and political decisions from the past so that we can make every effort to mitigate a future influenza pandemic. Unfortunately, predicting pandemics is thought to be impossible at this time; there is no discernible pattern for the emergence of pandemic influenza viral strains. As you might remember from chapter 2, influenza pandemics have occurred at intervals ranging between 10 and 50 years ever since the sixteenth century, with varying severity and impact. In addition to our inability to predict a future pandemic, we also do not have the tools to prevent the emergence of influenza pandemics: it is a matter of when (not if) the next pandemic will occur. The viruses of future pandemics are already in the making with the continual reassorting and evolving gene segments of the influenza viruses that are found within the billions of wild waterfowl and other animal hosts.

Luckily, many medical advances have occurred since the pandemic of 1918. We now have an incredible amount of information about the flu virus. Flu vaccines are updated yearly and are recommended annually. Antiviral drugs can be used to treat the flu (or even prevent it if used as chemoprophylaxis). Antibiotics can cure secondary bacterial infections. Diagnostic tests can quickly identify cases of the flu, and medical services, such as critical care units and advanced mechanical ventilations devices, can be utilized if needed. Given this progress, is it even possible for a future pandemic to match the severity of the Spanish flu of 1918? Many experts think so. Our world population has grown threefold since 1918 (the world population in 2018 was 7.6 billion people compared to 1.8 billion people in 1918), and as the human population has grown, so has the number of pigs and chickens required to feed them. Global movement of people and goods has increased substantially. What, then, can we do if a future pandemic is unavoidable? How can we use our knowledge from prior pandemics to limit the potential catastrophic consequences of a pandemic in this day and age?

Global Collaboration for Pandemic Preparedness

Many of the problems identified by the GPMB in their annual report on global preparedness for health emergencies were due to insufficient national and local leadership, lack of data sharing and medical countermeasures, broken finance systems with insufficient international funding, and inadequate international coordination mechanisms. The consequences of such limitations can be deadly, and the GPMB has called for urgent actions to prepare the world for its next health emergency. WHO has readily admitted that we are better prepared than we ever have been for a global emergency, but still not prepared *enough*. They concur that collaboration is key to help mitigate the risk and impact of a pandemic, as well as to manage pandemic response and recovery. Some recent accomplishments in influenza pandemic preparedness by WHO include

- establishment of the Research and Development Blueprint to aid organizations in identifying research needs and to work with country partners to plan for and implement studies during influenza epidemics;
- adoption of a framework to improve pandemic influenza preparedness globally and support a more equitable response; this has allowed support of countries financially and technically to improve certain essential public health capacities and establish a virtual stockpile of pandemic influenza vaccines (currently estimated at more than 400 million doses);
- increased Global Influenza Surveillance and Response System to 151 laboratories in 115 countries, which has resulted in commendation for timely identification, assessment, and monitoring of influenza and other respiratory pathogens; and
- increased funding for research for epidemics and development of vaccines to stop future epidemics.

In addition, WHO has outlined a Global Influenza Strategy, the goal of which is to prevent seasonal influenza, to control the spread of influenza from animals to humans, and to prepare for the next influenza pandemic. They have published an updated checklist for pandemic influenza risk and impact management, outlining essential and desired planning actions that should be the priority of all national authorities, including our U.S. government. In brief, the primary components of this checklist are as follows:

Planning, Coordination, and Resources

Successful operations occur when individuals know their roles and responsibilities, understand how they fit into the overall plan and how to work together, and have the capacities and resources to implement the plan. Unfortunately, the majority of countries that report to WHO still do not have a national pandemic plan, and as of 2016, only one-third of countries were in compliance with new milestones that were created to improve their response capacity for public health emergencies.

Legal and Policy Issues

In an emergency situation, it may be necessary to overrule existing laws or individual human rights in order to implement measures that are in the best interests of community health. Examples are the enforcement of quarantine, use of privately owned buildings for health care facilities, off-license use of drugs, compulsory vaccination, and implementation of emergency shifts in essential services. Development of a legal framework ensures transparent assessment and authority, as well as coherence with relevant international laws.

Ethical Issues

Difficult choices have to be made in the midst of a pandemic in order to secure the best health outcomes for individuals, groups, and communities. Policy decisions may result in a conflict between the goal to protect the health of the population and respect for individual rights and freedoms. Identifying an ethical framework in advance can help ensure that vulnerable populations are not harmed and that adequate consideration is given to ethical issues even when rapid action is required.

Risk Communication and Community Engagement

Exchange of information/advice between authorities/experts and the people at risk during a pandemic is essential to enable communities to understand the health risks they face and to make it easier to implement actions to protect themselves.

Points of Entry

To slow the international spread of a pandemic influenza virus, staff and infrastructure at points of entry (airports, ports, and ground crossings of international entry and exit of travelers, cargo, and conveyances) must be prepared to detect and manage ill people and to refer them to public health services in a safe manner.

Travel Restrictions

Countries should follow WHO's advice regarding travel restrictions, which may be issued if it is deemed useful in delaying the spread of the pandemic virus, especially if used in conjunction with other public health measures.

Laboratories

It is essential to have access to laboratories with influenza virus diagnostic capacity to quickly confirm suspected human cases of a new influenza strain. In 2008, the CDC established the International Reagent Resource, which provides substances to labs around the world needed to identify influenza viruses. During the 2009 H1N1 pandemic, this resource provided necessary testing assays to labs *within two weeks* of the first new viral strain identification.

Seasonal Influenza Surveillance

This interpandemic surveillance generates information that can be used to plan appropriate influenza control and intervention measures, allocate health resources, make influenza case management recommendations, and signal early warning of unusual disease activity that might be the result of a novel viral strain.

Nonseasonal Influenza Surveillance

Nonseasonal influenza virus surveillance systems detect the emergence of strains that have the potential to start a pandemic. This information can then be used in the development of prepandemic vaccines; in the United States, these vaccines are stored (along with facemasks, antiviral drugs, and other materials) in the Strategic National Stockpile in case of a pandemic.

Outbreak Investigation

Timely investigation of unusual cases or clusters of respiratory illness is key to the early detection of a novel influenza virus.

Pandemic Surveillance

This surveillance verifies reports of sustained human-to-human transmission of a novel viral strain, followed by the subsequent geographic spread, disease trends, transmission intensity, impact on health care services, and changes in antigenicity and antiviral drug sensitivity.

Health Services

Health services, including management of facilities, personnel scheduling/education/safety, maintenance of medicines/supplies/devices, and capacities of morgues, must be kept functioning in order to properly treat patients with pandemic influenza and to maintain essential care, particularly for vulnerable groups such as children, pregnant women, the elderly, and people with chronic conditions. In the pandemic of 1918, it was universally agreed that the single variable that was most associated with influenza survival was good nursing care. Even without antiviral medications, nurses provided nutrition, rest, warmth, fluids, fresh air, a comforting presence, and consistency in protective isolation.

Medical Countermeasures

Implementation of aggressive seasonal influenza vaccination programs contributes to better pandemic preparedness, but countries also need to assess their capacity to produce or procure pandemic influenza vaccines, to obtain antiviral drugs in an emergency situation, and to have antibiotics in ready supply. Autopsies that were done on people who died during the 1918 pandemic showed that secondary bacterial pneumonia was often the principal cause of death; at the same time, many of these people showed evidence of rapid repair of the viral damage. This would suggest that early antibiotic use and quality intensive care might influence recovery. Given that uncomplicated influenza can rapidly progress to a complicated illness, research to identify early indicators of pending bacterial pneumonia is necessary and immediate hospitalization for critical care, including intravenous antibiotics and mechanical ventilation, should be readily available. In the United States, we have moderately effective influenza vaccines and a vaccine production model that takes about six months; this timeline has to be reduced in the setting of a pandemic. (During the 2009 H1N1 pandemic, the first doses of a vaccine did not become available in the United States until 26 weeks after the decision to produce a pandemic vaccine was made.) Globally, pandemic flu vaccine capacity was estimated to be 6.4 billion doses in 2015; this is not enough to cover even half of the world's population should two doses be required for protection. We also have vaccines against *Streptococcus pneumoniae*, but not against the other prominent pathogens that cause secondary bacterial pneumonia (*Staphylococcus aureus* or *Streptococcus pyogenes)*; these vaccines should be considered a priority, too.

Non-Pharmaceutical Interventions

People and communities need to take measures beyond vaccinations and antiviral drugs to slow the spread of disease in a pandemic; these interventions are the first line of defense as they are universally and immediately available. Thanks to a better understanding of the failures of the public health approaches during the pandemic of 1918 (as well as successes from other epidemics and pandemics), we now know that isolation can limit and slow the spread of pandemics. For example, during the influenza pandemic of 1918, people in remote locations were known to have successfully isolated themselves to prevent infection. However, U.S. military camps (where men lived in close quarters) demonstrated the highest rates of death due to the spread of bacteria that caused secondary pneumonia. In the future, a global public health effort to isolate people could potentially blunt the effect of the pandemic, allowing decreased spread and decreased illness (or even death) as vaccines are manufactured and distributed. Another benefit to isolation is that people with high risk for severe infection could be identified, and their exposure to influenza could be limited with home confinement and monitoring, along with use of preventative antiviral medications. Other non-pharmaceutical interventions include respiratory etiquette, hand hygiene, using face masks in community settings, and routine environmental cleaning of frequently touched surfaces and objects. An additional consideration to be taken into account when preparing for a pandemic is animal-to-human transmission risks. People should know to avoid wild birds, to have no contact with poultry that appears ill or is noted to be dead, and to not touch surfaces that have been contaminated with droppings from wild birds or poultry. Attempts to reduce risk for variant flu strains at animal fairs and markets should be made as well. The CDC has outlined the following recommendations to limit risk of infection at animal fairs:

- Anyone attending fairs where pigs are present should not eat, drink, or put anything in their mouth in pig barns or show arenas.
- No toys, pacifiers, cups, strollers, or similar items should be taken into the pig barns or show arenas.
- People should wash their hands often with soap and water before and after pig exposure.
- Anyone sick with symptoms that could be due to the flu should avoid attending the event at all.
- People at high risk for serious influenza complications (including children younger than five years of age, people who are older than 65 years of age, pregnant women, and people with chronic diseases and/or immunosuppression) should avoid pigs and swine barns altogether.
- Handlers should wear protective clothing, gloves, and mask that covers the mouth and nose if a sick pig is present.
- Pig owners should be educated about good stockmanship and animal care, including vaccination. Pigs should be monitored every day and a veterinarian called if a pig appears to be sick.

- Management strategies should be in place to reduce the emergence and spread of influenza among herds, including surveillance testing and consideration of a shorter swine exhibition period (not more than three days at a time). Pigs who test positive for swine influenza at fairs should be isolated immediately.

Essential Service Continuity

Clean water, sanitation, electricity, fire and police services, financial services, communication, and access to food must be maintained during a pandemic to ensure welfare and stability within a community.

Recovery

An all-of-society collaboration will be required between government, businesses, community organizations, and the public to recover from a pandemic, and recovery may need to occur even as ongoing preparedness activities are in motion due to the potential for second and third waves of a pandemic.

Research and Development

A pandemic situation creates unique opportunities for research and data collection to increase knowledge about the influenza virus, the disease it causes, and the effectiveness of public health measures.

Evaluation

Evaluation is an essential part of pandemic operations, as it provides valuable information about the effectiveness of pandemic preparedness, response and recovery activities, and resource allocations.

As countries around the globe continue to prepare for the next influenza pandemic, you should do your part, too: get the flu vaccine *every year*, wash your hands often, and stay home if you are ill.

Case Illustrations

UNCOMPLICATED SEASONAL INFLUENZA

Mr. Branson is a 47-year-old Caucasian male with a past medical history notable only for a broken arm when he was a teenager. He works at a fitness center as a trainer, and while he is at work, he is responsible for individual client training sessions, oversight of the aerobic fitness area, and cleanup duties. On Wednesday, January 24, during a typical work shift, he noticed that he had a headache. Shortly afterward, he also began to appreciate an ache in his lower back, and the larger muscles of his arms and legs seemed sore, too. Though Mr. Branson was a regular exerciser, he hadn't done any robust lifting of weights or extended workouts to explain the muscle pain. He finished his shift that day, but by the time he got home, he was so tired that he told his wife he didn't want any dinner and that he wanted to go to bed early. He changed into his pajamas and tucked himself into bed. Several hours later, he was woken up by a sense of chills. Once he was fully awake, he noticed he was having uncontrollable shaking, and his teeth were even chattering. He called to his wife.

Upon entering the room, his wife noticed that he looked really sick. As the chills subsided, she felt his forehead, and it was hot to the touch. She took his temperature with a thermometer, which registered a reading of 102.4 degrees Fahrenheit—he definitely had a fever. Mr. Branson also said his throat hurt, that he was coughing a bit, and that he was a little nauseated. After drinking a glass of water and taking acetaminophen, he went back to sleep. Upon awakening in the morning, Mr. Branson still felt unwell and decided to call his primary doctor. He was given a walk-in appointment for later that day. Mr. Branson called into work to let them know he was ill and wouldn't be coming in for his shift. Luckily, his colleagues were understanding of his situation and could cover his client appointments. They also reiterated their work policy that focuses on keeping their clients safe: if you're sick, you should stay home.

Upon arrival at his doctor's office, the nurse gave him a mask for his nose and mouth and then took him to an exam room. She checked his vital signs: he was feverish again, with a slightly high heart rate and breathing rate. His oxygen levels and blood pressure readings were normal. Dr. Alvarez quickly joined him in the exam room and reviewed his symptoms: fever, chills, sore throat, nausea, muscle aches, headache, and fatigue. He didn't have any shortness of breath, though he did have an occasional dry cough. She looked at his throat (minimally red but dry), felt his neck (no markedly swollen glands), and listened to his heart (regular heart rhythm but fast rate) and lungs (clear). She also felt his abdomen (no masses or pain) and checked his skin (warm to the touch but without rash or swelling). Dr. Alvarez knew that the community was experiencing a wave of seasonal influenza and that a patient presenting with the symptoms described by Mr. Branson was very likely to have the flu. She also knew that Mr. Branson worked at a fitness center where he came in contact with multiple clients and public equipment during every shift, which would have put him at risk for exposure to the influenza virus. She asked Mr. Branson if he had gotten a flu shot that season; he said that he had hardly ever been sick in the past, so it just didn't seem like he would need it. She also asked him how often he washed his hands while at work; he sheepishly admitted that he occasionally used the alcohol-based gel but that he hardly ever stopped to wash with soap and water unless he used the restroom.

Dr. Alvarez told Mr. Branson that she thought he had the flu and that she didn't feel further diagnostic testing would be required to prove that diagnosis. Because he had been sick for less than 48 hours, she said he was a candidate for antiviral treatment; he was willing to take the medication, so she gave him a prescription for oseltamivir 75 mg to be taken by mouth twice a day for five days. Mr. Branson asked if there were any over-the-counter medications that would help him feel better, and Dr. Alvarez said that antipyretics, sore throat and cough suppressants, and anti-inflammatory medications might all help alleviate some of his symptoms. She also told him to drink enough liquids to stay hydrated and to cover his nose and mouth when sneezing or coughing. She agreed that he should stay home from work until he went 24 hours without a fever without taking any antipyretics. She reminded him that he should get a flu shot *every year*. Mr. Branson returned home and went to bed. After two days, he no longer had evidence of fevers, his sore throat and muscle pains were gone, and he felt fairly well rested. He was able to return to work for his next scheduled shift on Monday, though he noticed a residual cough for another week or two.

Analysis

Mr. Branson's presentation is quite classic for uncomplicated seasonal influenza: he had acute onset of symptoms, and his most prominent complaints were very typical for the flu, including fever, chills, aches and pains, sore throat, cough, and fatigue. During a seasonal influenza outbreak, people who have these symptoms have a very high likelihood of having the flu, and diagnostic testing is not necessarily needed as the treatment can easily be outlined. Mr. Branson had symptoms for less than 48 hours at the time of his office visit, so he was within the recommended window to receive antiviral medication, along with recommendations for supportive care. Dr. Alvarez was also right to tell Mr. Branson that he should plan to get a flu vaccination every year.

INFLUENZA DURING PREGNANCY RESULTING IN ACUTE VIRAL PNEUMONIA

Monica is a 29-year-old Black female who is 26 weeks pregnant with her first child. Though she was troubled by morning sickness early on, she has had a relatively uncomplicated pregnancy so far. She works full-time, and due to her busy schedule (including fairly frequent overtime at work), she has missed a couple of her routine pregnancy appointments at her obstetrician's office. On Saturday evening, December 21, Monica was at the mall trying to finish her Christmas shopping when she began to feel really tired. She went to the food court to grab a beverage and rest for a bit, but that didn't seem to help. She decided to head back home, promising to go to bed early, but while driving, she started to feel hot and sweaty. When she got home, she immediately took off her shoes and went to lie down on the couch. Her husband, surprised to see her home so quickly from shopping, came over to talk with her. He felt her forehead and noticed it was hot and her skin was wet. She also was breathing hard. He brought her a glass of orange juice and a blanket. Monica quickly fell asleep, and he went into the den to watch TV, where he promptly fell asleep. Upon awakening the next morning, he came out to check on Monica. She was still asleep on the couch, but she was breathing very fast and shallow. Her skin felt cold and clammy to the touch, but she was sweaty, too. She coughed intermittently, but she didn't wake up, even when he loudly called her name and rubbed her arm. He called 911, and Monica was taken to the nearest emergency department.

When Monica arrived at the ED, she was able to be aroused, but she was not very alert. Her vital signs showed a slightly low temperature reading, an elevated respiratory and heart rate, and low oxygen levels. On examination, the doctors noticed labored breathing with some crackling sounds from her lungs and a very fast heart rate. Her fingers and toes felt cold to the touch. An x-ray of her chest showed abnormalities in both lungs, and an influenza swab taken from her nasal passages quickly returned with a positive result. She was started on the antiviral medication oseltamivir. Despite this, Monica began to show more and more trouble with her breathing rate, and she was unable to keep her oxygen levels within the desired range. After her husband gave his consent, Monica had a breathing tube placed, and mechanical ventilation was started to aid in her breathing efforts. Her blood pressure dropped so low that she needed medications to boost it toward normal levels and allow adequate blood flow and oxygen to her vital organs, brain, and baby. She was transferred to the intensive care unit, where an interdisciplinary team of providers provided recommendations for care.

Monica required breathing assistance for almost two weeks, but she slowly was able to be weaned off the ventilator. Her medical team, including doctors specializing in intensive care, pulmonary medicine (lung specialists), infectious diseases, and high-risk obstetrics, monitored her clinical course closely in order to save both her and her baby. Monica was lucky—she survived her illness and she didn't lose her baby, but any influences on fetal development remain to be seen as she continues to delivery. Monica was so debilitated by her illness that she required a stay at a rehabilitation unit for an additional 10 days before she could be discharged to home.

Analysis

Monica's influenza illness was rapid in onset and notably severe, which is exactly the concern for pregnant women who become infected with the influenza virus. Pregnant and early postpartum women are known to be at risk for more severe disease and more worrisome outcomes, such as acute viral pneumonia, than nonpregnant women. Because Monica missed several of her routine pregnancy appointments, both she and her providers never realized that she had not been vaccinated against the flu. Her husband also had not been vaccinated, and he had been ill with upper respiratory symptoms the week before Monica became sick. Both Monica and her husband vowed to get their flu shot every year and promised that their child would be vaccinated, too. Monica and her baby were both very lucky. Acute viral pneumonia is a severe complication of influenza infection and there is a risk of death with this diagnosis. Indeed, it is now thought that one of the reasons that so many people died during the influenza pandemic of 1918 is because the H1N1 strain was likely to have caused acute viral pneumonia.

COMPLICATED INFLUENZA AND CHRONIC DISEASE

Fred is a 55-year-old Caucasian male with a past medical history of emphysema, which is a form of chronic lung disease that makes expelling air difficult. He was a known user of tobacco: he began smoking cigarettes when he was 15 and continued to smoke two packs a day until just last year. His lung problems have progressed to the point where he needs oxygen at home, and he is no longer able to work at the factory job he held for many years. Though Fred is only middle aged, his lung doctors have told him that his emphysema is advanced and severe. His lung doctors also stressed the importance of vaccination to prevent respiratory infections, so he has been vaccinated against pneumonia and influenza.

On Sunday, November 13, Fred went to church with his family and then enjoyed a buffet lunch afterward. He felt fine until Tuesday afternoon, when he began to feel chilled despite the fact that his home thermostat registered 70 degrees Fahrenheit. Soon, his chills became so bad that he heard his own teeth chattering. He also began to have an ache in his back. He got up from his recliner and moved to his bed, where he quickly fell asleep. He woke up hours later in the middle of the night, drenched in sweat and short of breath. As he got up from bed to use the bathroom, he could tell his breathing was off; he was really winded by the time he got back to bed. Using his portable bedside oxygen monitor, he found that he needed to increase the flow of his oxygen a bit. He decided that he would try to sleep until morning and then call his doctor for an appointment.

At the doctor's office, Fred was noted to have a fever, some respiratory distress with increased oxygen requirements, and a slightly high heart rate. Knowing it was flu season, his doctor elected to forego influenza testing and wrote a prescription for an antiviral medication targeting the flu. Fred stopped at the pharmacy on the drive home to fill the prescription, and he took his first dose upon arriving home. Then, he went back to bed. For the next few days, Fred took his prescribed antiviral medication as instructed, drank fluids to remain hydrated, slept often, and limited his activity to his house. By Friday, he was feeling much better—no further fevers, more energy, stable respiratory status, and a bit of a residual cough. But on Sunday morning as he was getting ready for church as usual, Fred felt hot and achy again. Puzzled by the return of symptoms, he took acetaminophen to reduce fever and pain. For the next two days, he had waxing and waning fevers, shaking chills, muscle aches, and progressively worsened breathing. He also started to cough up yellowish sputum flecked with blood. When he didn't show up for a Tuesday night family dinner, his niece dropped by his house to check on him. She found him lying in bed, and he didn't wake up when she called his name. She also noticed that he was clearly having trouble breathing. She called 911, and an ambulance took Fred directly to the hospital.

On arrival to the ED, he was found to have a fever, a fast heart rate, and an elevated respiratory rate that was associated with very labored breathing. He also couldn't seem to keep his oxygen levels or his blood pressure stable. With concern that his was heading toward dangerously low oxygen levels and impending respiratory failure, the ED doctors elected to place a breathing tube and to connect Fred to a breathing machine. Suspicious of septic shock, they took a sample of his sputum and his blood to look for evidence of infection—within 24 hours, all of the samples showed growth of a bacteria called *Staphylococcus aureus.* His chest x-ray was also abnormal with findings consistent with severe and invasive pneumonia. Over the course of the next few days, Fred showed rapid clinical deterioration. Despite the breathing assistance, use of antibiotics, and titration of medications to increase his blood pressure, Fred showed little improvement. Further imaging of his lungs was done, showing necrotic tissue with large cavitary lesions. On the seventh hospital day, Fred went into an abnormal heart rhythm. Though the ICU doctors tried to return his heart to a viable rhythm with use of special medications and shocks via a defibrillator, Fred was pronounced dead. Cause of death was noted to be influenza complicated by secondary bacterial pneumonia with septic shock and multisystem organ failure.

Analysis

Though it may seem surprising that people can still die of complications of influenza, it is, unfortunately, very true. Initially, Fred's clinical scenario was quite classic for seasonal flu, which can occur after vaccination due to viral strain mismatch. Fred sought medical attention and his doctor treated him appropriately for the likely diagnosis of influenza. Sadly, though, the recurrence of symptoms later in the week was a hint that Fred was likely to have a secondary bacterial infection—return of symptoms after an initial period of improvement with the flu should prompt medical attention, especially in a person with a chronic disease that puts them at high risk for severe complications of influenza. As can happen in the setting of a bacterial pneumonia, the infection spread from his lungs to his bloodstream and he rapidly became ill with septic shock and severe respiratory distress. In the setting of underlying chronic lung disease, Fred was unable to withstand the attack of the virulent *Staphylococcus* bacteria. The ED and ICU providers did everything possible to keep him alive, but the infection overwhelmed his already diseased lungs and, ultimately, caused his heart to fail.

COMPLICATED INFLUENZA IN A YOUNG CHILD

Dora is a four-year-old Hispanic female who has a past medical history of ear infections, though she hasn't been ill much this year. Dora's mom works at a nursing home, so she attends preschool in the morning and day care in the afternoon until her mom can pick her up after work. She loves the day care center—she has lots of friends, an unending supply of toys, and a delicious lunch when she arrives after school. On Friday, December 2, when Dora got to day care, she noticed her best friend Alexander wasn't there. The day care attendant told her that Alex was sick and resting at home. That night, at dinner, Mom noticed that Dora's cheeks looked a bit flushed and that she hadn't eaten much off her plate. She felt Dora's forehead, and it was hot to the touch. She got a thermometer to confirm, and yes, Dora had a fever. Her mom gave her a medicine to bring down the fever. Dora lay on the couch while her mom watched television, and within minutes, she was asleep. When they were ready to go to bed, Mom carried her into her bedroom and tucked her underneath the quilt.

The next morning, Mom woke up first to her alarm. She was surprised that Dora wasn't already up, since she often jumped into her bed to say good morning. She went to Dora's room, and before she even made it past the doorway, she could hear loud and unusual breathing noises. Every time Dora took a breath in, she made a high-pitched noise, and though she was still asleep, she coughed often. The cough was harsh in tone, and it reminded Mom of the barking seals at the zoo. Dora seemed to be breathing fast, and she was sweaty and flushed. Mom called the pediatrician's answering service to see if she should bring Dora in for an appointment.

Dr. Watts called back quickly even though it was still early morning and the clinic wasn't open yet. She listened to the description of the fever and poor appetite the night before and the development of loud breathing noises and cough overnight. She asked Mom to put the phone next to Dora's mouth so that she could hear the noises for herself. Immediately, she recognized the symptoms of croup. Concerned about Dora's abnormal breathing pattern and her unwillingness to wake for food or drink, Dr. Watts suggested to Mom that she bring Dora to the emergency room for evaluation. Mom needed to be at work in just 45 minutes, and she didn't have paid sick or family leave. How could she handle a sick kid who needed to go to the ED? Mom called her employer first; luckily, after a bit of explanation and negotiation, she was given permission to take the day off, but without pay. Dora woke up as her mom was getting her ready to go to the ED. She was irritable and started to cry, which made her breathing and cough sound even worse. She didn't want anything to eat or drink, and she didn't even have to use the bathroom.

Upon arrival to the ED, Dora immediately had an IV started, and she was given intravenous fluids. A quick swab of her nasal passages was performed to test for infection, and she was started on a special breathing treatment with oxygen and adrenaline. Within an hour, Dora looked and sounded better—her breathing was less rapid and not quite as noisy, and she asked if she could have something to drink. The ED doctor came back to check on her and told Mom that the influenza A test was positive and that her daughter's croup was a result of the flu. Within several more hours, Dora had improved enough to go home. Mom was handed the discharge paperwork, which included prescriptions for an antiviral medication and steroids.

Dora steadily improved, and within three days, she was back to normal health. Mom found out that Alex had also been diagnosed with the flu but that he didn't suffer from any symptoms of croup. Though Dora came through her illness just fine, Mom started to feel unwell about two days after Dora's ED visit, and she was also found to have the flu. Because she worked in a nursing home, she was told to stay home until she had no fever for 24 hours without use of any antipyretics. Mom had to miss work for an additional three days, all without pay.

Analysis

It has been estimated that 15–42 percent of preschool and school-aged children become infected with influenza each year, and these infections are associated with an increased number of outpatient health care visits, increased rates of hospitalization, more absences from school for both the child and their siblings, and many missed workdays for parents. Certainly, in Dora's case, her influenza infection caused more complications than just a simple upper respiratory infection. She had manifestations consistent with croup, required an ED evaluation, and caused almost a week away from work without pay for her mother. Even though Dora completed a course of an antiviral medication, her mom got the flu, too. This is not completely unexpected since children are highly contagious with influenza and can shed virus for days (Mom was employed by a nursing home, so contact with residents and other employees at the home also put her at risk for exposure to influenza). Presumptively, Dora was exposed to the virus by her infected best friend at day care. The pediatrician was appropriate in quickly assessing the clinical situation and sending Dora to the ED for evaluation given the respiratory symptoms, the lethargy, and the lack of desire to eat and drink without normal urination. The ED staff was prompt in their assessment and treatment for the croup.

UNCOMPLICATED INFLUENZA WITH VACCINATION CONCERNS

Shandrah is an 18-year-old Indo-American female who is a freshman at State University. She thoroughly enjoys college life and has just decided to study nursing. Shandrah's parents are both professors at the university; her mom teaches psychology and her dad does research in the geology lab. Growing up, Shandrah's parents felt that the childhood vaccination schedule was overwhelming and were concerned about all of the questionable safety issues related to vaccines that they read about online. Despite pleas by her pediatrician to consider vaccination, Shandrah's parents refused the injections at each clinic visit. Shandrah had a fairly normal health history growing up: she had the occasional upper respiratory infection, and she broke her arm after falling off a skateboard when she was seven. Luckily, she never became ill with any of the germs that the childhood vaccines were meant to prevent.

On Friday, January 14, after her 8:00 a.m. class, Shandrah noticed that she felt slightly dizzy when going down the stairs. She also felt uncomfortably warm and her muscles hurt, almost like she had worked out really hard the day before. She decided to skip the rest of her morning classes and headed back to her dorm room. Her roommate was there and commented that her cheeks looked flushed and that her voice seemed slightly hoarse. Shandrah changed back into her pajamas and lay in bed. Though she had been warm on her way back to her room, she suddenly became cold and began shaking with chills. Her mouth seemed dry and her throat hurt; she also seemed to have a "catch" in her throat, and she kept wanting to cough. The symptoms waxed and waned throughout the night, and the next morning, her roommate convinced her to go to the Student Clinic.

When they checked her temperature at the clinic, it was almost 102 degrees Fahrenheit. Her heart rate was elevated, too. The triage nurse knew that influenza was prevalent on campus, and she immediately swabbed Shandrah's nose to send off a rapid flu test. It came back positive for influenza B. The clinic doctor entered the room and did a brief examination. She told Shandrah about the positive flu test and said she would write a prescription for an antiviral medication that would hopefully limit the severity and duration of her symptoms. She asked Shandrah if she'd had the flu vaccination that year, and Shandrah admitted that her parents had refused all vaccines up to that point. Noting that Shandrah seemed embarrassed by this, the doctor asked Shandrah about her thoughts on vaccination. Shandrah mentioned that she'd done some reading and that she wasn't sure she agreed with her parents, especially because she was hoping to become a nurse one day. She felt that vaccines were safe, that they were effective, and that they were a major achievement in the world of medicine. She also said that as a future nurse, it seemed unethical not to protect herself and her future patients against communicable diseases. The doctor nodded her head and said, "Shandrah, you're exactly right—it's amazing that you've come to that conclusion about vaccination all on your own. At your age, you can make your own decisions about vaccinations. Once you're over your bout with the flu, come back to the clinic, and we can talk about a vaccine schedule for you."

Analysis

Shandrah's symptoms were consistent with a classic case of uncomplicated influenza, which can be caused by either A or B flu strains (the physical symptoms are indistinguishable between the strains). The triage nurse was quick to recognize the presentation as likely influenza, and the rapid test confirming the diagnosis was done quickly. The doctor offered appropriate therapy. It is unknown if Shandrah could have avoided influenza had she been vaccinated earlier in the season. What is clear, however, is that Shandrah is at risk for many other infectious diseases beyond influenza, and her lack of vaccination offers no herd immunity to her roommates or fellow college students. Luckily, Shandrah is thoughtful, intelligent, and interested in both her own and others' health. Despite her parents' misperceptions about vaccines, she has realized that they are safe, effective, and beneficial. She has also recognized that her future job as a nurse comes with a moral commitment to protect the health of her patients. The clinic doctor was empathetic and willing to talk to Shandrah about vaccinations. Hopefully, she will take all she has learned about vaccines home to discuss further with her parents so that they can also become advocates for vaccination.

Glossary

Acute phase
Term referring to the first several weeks of an illness before antibody responses are maximized.

Acute Respiratory Distress Syndrome (ARDS)
Clinical condition of the lungs often resulting in respiratory failure caused by disintegration of tissue during a host's immune response to an infection.

Adsorption
Process in which HA binds to sialic acid found on the surface of respiratory tract epithelial cells in order to gain entry into the cells.

Antibody
Protein product of the immune system, which neutralizes or destroys infectious agents.

Antigen
Any substance foreign to the body that is capable of binding with a product of the immune system, allowing an immune response to occur.

Antigenic drift
Genetic mutations occurring at antigenic sites on the hemagglutinin and neuraminidase proteins of the influenza viral particle.

Antigenic shift
Mutations that arise from a cross of animal and human viral strains with drastic alterations in the HA and NA structures, resulting in an entirely novel virus.

Antipyretics
Medications that are used to reduce fever, such as acetaminophen or ibuprofen.

Arrhythmia
Abnormal heart rhythm.

Arthralgia
Joint pain, which is a common manifestation during illness with the flu.

Attenuation
Alteration of a virus so that it is weakened, less virulent, and unable to cause actual infection.

Biphasic fever curve
Return of fever days after an infection appears to have already been resolved.

Blood generation theory
Belief that a spontaneous chemical process in the blood can make people sick.

Bronchus
Either of the two primary divisions of the trachea that lead into the right and left lungs.

Cardiac tamponade
Compression of the heart due to the accumulation of fluid within its lining.

CD4 cells
Specific type of T lymphocyte that helps with generation of antibodies and activation of cytokines in response to infection.

CD8 cells
Specific type of T lymphocyte that helps kill host cells that have been invaded by an infectious agent.

Cellular immunity
The pathway of the immune system that protects against an infectious agent using white blood cells.

Centrifuge
A machine that allows separation of substances using centrifugal force.

Chemoprophylaxis
Use of medications in an attempt to prevent infection.

Cilia
Projections from respiratory epithelial cells, which continuously beat in a sweeping motion.

Cohorting
Placing patients with the same infection in a shared hospital room.

Conjunctiva
Mucous membrane that lines the eyelids and eye.

Conjunctivitis
Inflammation of the conjunctiva.

Convalescent phase
A period of time beyond an infection when antibody response can best be detected in the blood.

Cyanosis
A lack of oxygen in vital tissues that results in a bluish discoloration, which often can be best seen in the lips, fingers, and toes.

Cytokines
Specific substances triggered by the immune system in response to infection.

Deoxyribonucleic acid (DNA)
Strand of genes that encode proteins, made up of deoxyribose sugars, phosphates, and four bases (adenine, guanine, cytosine, and thymine).

Elemental theory
The belief that everything is composed of four elements (water, earth, air, and fire), and that these elements are moved by two opposing forces (love and strife).

Emanate
To come out from a source.

Empathy
The ability to recognize and understand the feelings, thoughts, and experiences of someone else.

Endonuclease
An enzyme that breaks down the internal covalent bonds between nucleotides.

Epidemic
An outbreak that is confined to one location, such as a city or a country.

False-negative
A negative test result despite the presence of the disease or infection.

False-positive
A positive test result despite a lack of the disease or infection.

Fecal-oral
Route of germ transmission whereby a host comes in contact with fecal matter and then transmits the germ, hiding in the fecal matter, to their mouth.

Flow murmur
An atypical sound heard through the stethoscope as blood moves quickly and forcefully past the heart valves.

Germ theory
Belief that pathogens cause infectious diseases, even if they can't be seen by the naked eye.

Glycolipids
A type of lipid that also contains a carbohydrate portion.

Glycoproteins
A class of proteins that have carbohydrate groups attached.

Hemagglutination
The clumping together of red blood cells.

Hemagglutinin (HA)
A glycoprotein antigenic site projecting from the influenza viral envelope, which allows attachment of the virus to the cell of a host.

Herald wave
A brief spike in cases caused by an entirely new strain of flu at the end of an epidemic.

Herd immunity
Stopping the spread of a contagious disease through a population by achieving a high proportion of individual immunity, especially through vaccination.

Humidifier
A machine that expels tiny drops of water into the air, allowing for extra moisture that can help ease breathing.

Humoral immunity
The pathway of the immune system that protects against an infectious agent through production of antibodies.

Ill humor theory
The belief that ill humors result when water, earth, air, and fire enter the body through food, drink, and the atmosphere.

Immunity
A state in which a host is protected against a specific infectious agent.

Immunogenicity
The ability of a vaccine to produce a protective immune response.

Immunosenescence
The gradual deterioration of the body's immune system response with age.

Incubation period
The time period between infection with a pathogen and onset of identifiable symptoms.

Inoculate
To introduce material into another to promote growth or stimulate the immune system.

Miasma theory
The belief that the air could become infested with a contagious influence when combined with the decomposing organic matter from the earth.

Mitigate
To make less severe.

Morbidity
A diseased state manifesting in symptoms of ill health.

Mortality
The death of large numbers of people.

Myalgia
Muscle ache, a common manifestation during illness with influenza.

Myocarditis
Inflammation of the heart muscle.

Myositis
Inflammation of the muscles.

Neuraminidase (NA)
A glycoprotein antigenic site projecting from the influenza viral envelope, which allows full penetration of the virus into a host cell and separation from the host cell after replication.

Nucleotides
A unit of RNA or DNA composed of a nitrogenous base, a sugar, and a phosphate.

Outbreak
Occurrence of a large number of cases of influenza in a short period of time.

Pandemic
Progression of an influenza outbreak over a wide geographic area, affecting an exceptionally high proportion of the population, resulting in extraordinary morbidity and mortality.

Pathogen
A specific infectious agent that causes disease.

Patient etiquette
Appropriate behaviors when visiting a medical provider to improve rapport and aid in more accurate diagnosis and treatment outcomes.

Pericardial effusion
Collection of fluid surrounding the heart.

Pericarditis
Inflammation of the lining of the heart.

Placebo
A preparation designed to look like medicine but is pharmacologically inert.

Plasmapheresis
A process of removing the plasma from a sick person and replacing it with either plasma or high-dose antibodies from healthy donors.

Pleurisy
Pain at the chest experienced with deep breathing due to inflammation of the lining of the lungs.

Pneumonia
An acute inflammation of lung tissue and clogging of the air sacs with white blood cells and debris due to infection.

Polymerase
An enzyme that allows formation of RNA or DNA using preexisting DNA or RNA as a template.

Primary viral pneumonia
An infection in the lungs caused by the influenza virus itself.

Rebound congestion
Expansion of the tiny blood vessels in the nose that occurs with excessive use of decongestant nasal sprays.

Replication
Use of a viral genome to produce more viral particles.

Reverse evolution
A process of backward evolution that has been proposed as an explanation for the origin of viruses.

Rhabdomyolysis
Destruction of muscle tissue with release of the breakdown products into the bloodstream, sometimes leading to acute kidney injury.

Ribonucleic acid (RNA)
Strand of genes that encode proteins, made up of ribose sugars, phosphates, and four bases (adenine, guanine, cytosine, and uracil).

Rule utilitarianism
The ideology that a rule for society should be established that has the best outcome for the greatest number of people in the society.

Secondary bacterial pneumonia
Pneumonia caused by a bacteria that can occur concurrently (or shortly after) infection with influenza.

Sequestration
Ability of proteins encoded by the influenza virus to hide the viral RNA.

Serological testing
Laboratory testing of blood for evidence of antibodies, which can signify prior infection with the flu.

Soluble
Able to be dissolved in a liquid.

Subcutaneous emphysema
Pockets of air that accumulate just beneath the skin, often giving a crackling sound when pressed.

T lymphocytes
A type of white blood cell which participates in the host immune response.

Transcription
Process of copying DNA into a complementary RNA before proteins can be produced.

Translation
Production of proteins from the genetic code found in RNA.

Vaccination
Administration of low levels of an attenuated or deactivated infectious agent (or an agent so similar that it can "trick" the body) in order to produce antibodies for future protection against the infection.

Vaccine hesitancy
An attitude that is characterized by concern that vaccines should perhaps not be administered despite scientific evidence of their efficacy and safety.

Variolation
A technique in which pus or scabs taken from active smallpox (a disease caused by a virus named variola) are rubbed into the skin of another.

Viral shedding
Detection of viral particles in the respiratory secretions of a host infected with influenza.

Virion
A viral particle.

Virulence
Ability of a pathogen to overcome bodily defense mechanisms to cause a rapid, severe, and destructive course.

Zoonotic
An infection or disease that is transmissible from animals to humans.

Directory of Resources

BOOKS

Barry JM. 2004. *The Great Influenza: The Epic Story of the Deadliest Plague in History.* New York: Viking.

Crosby AW. 2003. *America's Forgotten Pandemic: The Influenza of 1918*, 2nd ed. New York: Cambridge University Press.

Davies P. 2000. *The Devil's Flu: The World's Deadliest Influenza Epidemic and the Scientific Hunt for the Virus that Caused It.* New York: Henry Holt and Company.

Garrett L. 1994. *The Coming Plague: Newly Emerging Diseases in a World Out of Balance.* New York: Farrar, Straus, and Giroux.

Karlen A. 1995. *Man and Microbes: Disease and Plagues in History and Modern Times.* New York: G.P. Putnam & Sons.

Kolata G. 1999. *Flu: The Story of the Great Influenza Pandemic of 1918 and the Search for the Virus That Caused It.* New York: Simon & Schuster.

HEALTH INFORMATION FOR THE PUBLIC

Centers for Disease Control and Prevention (CDC)
cdc.gov/flu/index.htm
Considered the nation's health protection agency, the CDC was created to protect America from health and safety threats, both foreign and domestic. The CDC website offers extensive information on the flu for the general public, including influenza activity and surveillance, prevention, symptoms and diagnosis, and treatment.

Medline Plus Health Information
medlineplus.gov/flu.html

Medline Plus Health Information is an online site under the umbrella of the U.S. National Library of Medicine, and it offers information about influenza (and other diseases, conditions, and wellness issues) in an easy-to-read language that everyone can understand.

National Foundation for Infectious Diseases (NFID)
nfid.org/infectious-diseases/influenza-flu/
The NFID's website is designed to provide education to the public and health care professionals about the burden, causes, prevention, diagnosis, and treatment of infectious diseases (including influenza) across the life span.

NIH Medline Plus Magazine
magazine.medlineplus.gov/topic/flu/
This online magazine is an official website of the U.S. government and is under the auspices of the National Institutes of Health (NIH) and the U.S. National Library of Medicine. It provides reliable, trusted, and up-to-date information on health topics, such as influenza, as well as updates on the latest breakthroughs from NIH-supported research.

WebMD
webmd.com/cold-and-flu/default.htm
The WebMD site uses a team of over 100 nationwide doctors and health experts across a broad range of specialty areas to provide credible information, supportive communities, and in-depth reference materials about health subjects, such as the flu.

World Health Organization (WHO)
int/en/news-room/fact-sheets/detail/influenza-(seasonal)
WHO is a global health organization whose primary role is to direct international health within the United Nations' system and to lead partners in global health responses. While WHO's website can be a source of information for emerging health issues all over the world, it also offers data, fact sheets, publications, and FAQs on many health topics, including influenza, for the general public.

HEALTH INFORMATION FOR MEDICAL PROVIDERS

Bookshelf
ncbi.nim.nih.gov/books
A resource of the National Center for Biotechnology Information (NCBI), under the umbrella of the NIH and the U.S. National Library of

Medicine, the Bookshelf website provides free online access to books and documents in life science and health care.

Centers for Disease Control and Prevention (CDC)
cdc.gov/flu/professionals/index.htm
Considered the nation's health protection agency, the CDC was created to protect America from health and safety threats, both foreign and domestic. Though the CDC website offers extensive information about the flu for the general public, it also has specific pages geared toward the needs of health professionals, including clinical evaluation and diagnosis, antiviral drugs, infection control, and influenza vaccination.

Infectious Diseases Society of America (IDSA)
idsociety.org/journals--publications/journals--publications-landing/
The IDSA is a community of over 12,000 physicians, scientists, and public health experts who specialize in infectious disease with a purpose of improving the health of individuals, communities, and society by promoting excellence in patient care, education, research, public health, and prevention related to infectious diseases such as influenza. Through the IDSA website, health care professionals can access journals, relevant news, an open discussion forum, and clinical practice guidelines.

Medscape
medscape.com
Medscape is an online destination for physicians and health care professionals worldwide, offering the latest medical news and expert perspectives, essential point-of-care drug and disease information, and relevant professional education.

PubMed
ncbi.nim.nih.gov/pubmed
PubMed is a government website through the NCBI, NIH, and U.S. National Library of Medicine that offers more than 28 million citations for biomedical literature from Medline, life science journals, and online books.

World Health Organization (WHO)
who.int/influenza/en/
The WHO is a global health organization whose primary role is to direct international health within the United Nations' system and to lead partners in global health responses. While the WHO's website can be used as a source of information about influenza for the general

public, it also offers material regarding influenza surveillance, the global influenza strategy, and pandemic preparedness that may be a resource for interested health care providers.

SPECIFIC INFLUENZA WEBSITES

Families Fighting Flu
familiesfightingflu.org
Families Fighting Flu is a nonprofit organization that works to educate others about the dangers of influenza and the critical importance of annual flu vaccination.

Flu Near You
flunearyou.org
Created by epidemiologists at Harvard, Boston Children's Hospital, and The Skoll Global Threats Fund, Flu Near You is a website that tracks voluntary reporting of flu symptoms, which are analyzed in order to generate local and national maps of influenza-like illness.

VACCINE INFORMATION

Immunization Action Coalition
immunize.org/influenza/
The Immunization Action Coalition is a nonprofit organization that works to increase immunization rates and prevent disease by creating and distributing educational materials that enhance delivery of safe and effective immunization services and by facilitating communication about the safety, efficacy, and use of vaccines between patients, parents, health care organizations, and government health agencies.

U.S. Department of Health and Human Services (HHS)
vaccines.gov/diseases/flu
This HHS website offers reliable, easy-to-understand information from the federal government of the United States on vaccines, immunizations, and vaccine-preventable diseases.

Vaccine Adverse Event Reporting System (VAERS)
vaers.hhs.gov
VAERS is a national vaccine safety surveillance program, run by the CDC and FDA, that strives to (a) detect new, unusual, or rare adverse events that happen after vaccination, (b) monitor increases in known

side effects, (c) identify potential patient risk factors for particular types of health problems related to vaccines, (d) assess the safety of newly licensed vaccines, (e) watch for unexpected or unusual patterns in adverse event reports, and (f) serve as a monitoring system in public health emergencies.

Vaccine Injury Compensation Program (VICP)
benefits.gov/benefit/641
The VICP, run by the Health Resources and Services Administration, was created after the political and financial fallout from the 1976 Swine flu vaccination plan. It compensates people whose injuries may have been caused by certain vaccines.

Bibliography

Andrewes CH. 1956. "Influenza: Theme and Variations." *California Medicine* 84:375–380.

Andrewes CH. 1973. "Fifty Years with Viruses." *Annual Review of Microbiology* 27:1–14.

Barberis I, Myles P, et al. 2016. "History and Evolution of Influenza Control Through Vaccination: From the First Monovalent Vaccine to Universal Vaccines." *Journal of Preventative Medicine and Hygiene* 57(3):e115–e120.

Barry JM. 2004. *The Great Influenza: The Epic Story of the Deadliest Plague in History.* New York: Viking.

Bates B. 1991. *A Guide to Physical Examination and History Taking,* 5th ed. Philadelphia: J.B. Lippincott Company.

Beckman HB and Frankel RM. 1984. "The Effect of Physician Behavior on the Collection of Data." *Annals of Internal Medicine* 102:520–528.

Beveridge WIB. 1977. *Influenza: The Last Great Plague.* New York: Prodist, Neale Watson Academic Publications.

Black M and Armstrong P. 2006. "An Introduction to Avian and Pandemic Influenza." *New South Wales Public Health Bulletin* 17(7–8):99–103.

Blaser MJ. 2006. "Pandemics and Preparations." *Journal of Infectious Diseases* 194:S70–S72.

Bureau of Public Affairs Fact Sheet. 2007. *U.S. Government Support to Combat Avian and Pandemic Influenza—An Update.* https://2001-2009.state.gov/r/pa/scp/2008/111243.htm

Centers for Disease Control and Prevention. 2019a. *Influenza: Information for Health Professionals.* https://www.cdc.gov/flu/professionals/index.htm

Centers for Disease Control and Prevention. 2019b. *Vaccines & Immunizations.* https://www.cdc.gov/vaccines/

Chattopadhyay I, Kiciman E, et al. 2018. *Conjunction of Factors Triggering Waves of Seasonal Influenza.* eLIFE. https://elifesciences.org/articles/30756

Cox NJ and Subbarao K. 2000. "Global Epidemiology of Influenza: Past and Present." *Annual Reviews of Medicine* 51:407–421.

Crosby AW. 2003. *America's Forgotten Pandemic: The Influenza of 1918,* 2nd ed. New York: Cambridge University Press.

Davies P. 2000. *The Devil's Flu: The World's Deadliest Influenza Epidemic and the Scientific Hunt for the Virus that Caused It.* New York: Henry Holt and Company.

Dehner G. 2012. *Influenza: A Century of Science and Public Health Response.* UPCC Book Collections on Project MUSE. Pittsburgh, PA: University of Pittsburgh Press. http://search.ebscohost.com/login.aspx?direct=true&AuthType=ip,shib&db=nlebk&AN=829348&site=eds–live&scope=site

Devlin RK. 2008. *Influenza.* Westport, CT: Greenwood Press.

Diamond J. 1998. *Guns, Germs and Steel: A Short History of Everybody for the Last 13000 Years.* London: Vintage.

Ebell MH, White LL, et al. 2004. "A Systematic Review of the History and Physical Examination to Diagnose Influenza." *Journal of the American Board of Family Physicians* 17:1–5.

Fauci AS. 2006. "Seasonal and Pandemic Influenza Preparedness: Science and Countermeasures." *Journal of Infectious Diseases* 194:S73–S76.

Fernandez E. 2002. *The Virus Detective: Dr. John Hultin Has Found Evidence of the 1918 Flu Epidemic That Has Eluded Experts for Decades.* http:/www.sfgate.com/cgi–bin/article.cgi?file=/chronicle/archive/2002/02/17/CM40502.DTL

Fiore AE, Shay DK, et al. 2007. "Prevention and Control of Influenza: Recommendations of the Advisory Committee on Immunization Practices (ACIP), 2007." *MMWR Recommendations and Reports* 56:1–54.

Frances ME, King ML, et al. 2019. "Back to the Future for Influenza Preimmunity—Looking Back at Influenza Virus History to Infer the Outcome of Future Infections." *Viruses* 11(2):122.

García-Sastre A and Whitley RJ. 2006. "Lessons Learned from Reconstructing the 1918 Influenza Pandemic." *Journal of Infectious Diseases* 194:S127–S132.

Garrett L. 1994. *The Coming Plague: Newly Emerging Diseases in a World Out of Balance.* New York: Farrar, Straus, and Giroux.

Global Preparedness Monitoring Board. 2019. *A World at Risk: Annual Report on Global Preparedness for Health Emergencies.* Geneva: World Health Organization.

Gottleib S. 2018. "FDA Approves Xofluza as First New Flu Treatment in Nearly 20 Years." *Infectious Disease News* 31(12):18.

Groom AV, Hennessy TW, et al. 2014. "Pneumonia and Influenza Mortality Among American Indian and Alaska Native People, 1990–2009." *American Journal of Public Health* 104(Suppl 3):S460–S469.

Hayden FG and Pavia AT. 2006. "Antiviral Management of Seasonal and Pandemic Influenza." *Journal of Infectious Diseases* 194:S127–S132.

Hays JN. 1998. *The Burdens of Disease: Epidemics and Human Response in Western History.* New Brunswick, NJ: Rutgers University Press.

Heymann DL. 2015. "Influenza." In: *Control of Communicable Diseases Manual,* 20th ed. Washington, DC: American Public Health Association, pp. 306–322.

Hussain A, Ali S, et al. 2018. "The Anti-Vaccination Movement: A Regression in Modern Medicine." *Cureus* 10(7): e2919. https://www.cureus.com/articles/13250-the-anti-vaccination-movement-a-regression-in-modern-medicine

Iannelli V. 2019. "New Flu Virus Strains." *VeryWell Health.* https://www.verywellhealth.com/new-flu-virus-strains-2633828

Influenza Specialist Group. 2015. *About Influenza.* http://www.isg.org.au/index.php/about-influenza/

Institute of Medicine Forum on Microbial Threats. 2010. *Infectious Disease Movement in a Borderless World: Workshop Summary.* Washington DC: National Academies Press.

Karlen A. 1995. *Man and Microbes: Disease and Plagues in History and Modern Times.* New York: G.P. Putnam & Sons.

Kilbourne ED. 2006. "Influenza Pandemics of the 20th Century." *Emerging Infectious Diseases* 12(1):9–14.

Kolata G. 1999. *Flu: The Story of the Great Influenza Pandemic of 1918 and the Search for the Virus That Caused It.* New York: Simon & Schuster.

Korsch BM and Harding C. 1997. *The Intelligent Patient's Guide to the Doctor–Patient Relationship: Learning How to Talk So Your Doctor Will Listen.* New York: Oxford University Press.

Madhav N, Oppenheim B, et al. 2017. "Pandemics: Risks, Impacts, and Mitigation." In: *Disease Control Priorities: Improving Health and Reducing Poverty,* 3rd ed. (Jamison DT, Gelband H, et al., eds.). Washington, DC: International Bank for Reconstruction and Development/The World Bank.

Markowitz S, Nesson E, et al. 2019. "The Effects of Employment on Influenza Rates." *Economics & Human Biology* 34:286–295.

Martini M, Gazzaniga V, et al. 2019. "The Spanish Influenza Pandemic: A Lesson from History 100 Years After 1918." *Journal of Preventative*

Medicine and Hygiene 60(1):e64–e67. https://www.ncbi.nlm.nih.gov/pmc/articles/PMC6477554/

McConnell CP. 2000. "The Treatment of Influenza." *Journal of the American Osteopathic Association* 100:311–313.

McKee C and Bohannon K. 2016. "Exploring the Reasons Behind Parental Refusal of Vaccines." *Journal of Pediatric Pharmacology and Therapeutics* 21(2):104–109.

Moghadami M. 2017. "A Narrative Review of Influenza: A Seasonal and Pandemic Disease." *Iranian Journal of Medical Sciences* 42(1):2–13.

Molinari NAM, Ortega-Sanchez IR, et al. 2007. "The Annual Impact of Seasonal Influenza in the US: Measuring Disease Burden and Costs." *Vaccine* 25(27):5086–5096.

Morens DM and Taubenberger JK. 2006. "Influenza and the Origins of the Phillips Collection, Washington, DC." *Emerging Infectious Diseases* 12:78–80.

Morens DM and Taubenberger JK. 2018. "The Mother of All Pandemics is 100 Years Old (and Going Strong)!" *American Journal of Public Health* 108(11):1449–1454.

Morgan A. 2006. "Avian Influenza: An Agricultural Perspective." *Journal of Infectious Diseases* 194:S139–S146.

Morse SS, ed. 1993. *Emerging Viruses.* New York: Oxford University Press.

National Foundation for Infectious Diseases. 2019. "Survey: Most Adults Unaware of Flu Risks from Chronic Health Conditions." *Infectious Disease News* 32(1):34–35.

Nichol KL and Treanor JJ. 2006. "Vaccines for Seasonal and Pandemic Influenza." *Journal of Infectious Diseases* 194:S111–S118.

Nicholson KG, Webster RG, et al., eds. 1998. *Textbook of Influenza,* 1st ed. Oxford: Blackwell Science.

Nuwer R. 2018. *What If a Deadly Influenza Pandemic Broke Out Today?* BBC. http://www.bbc.com/future/story/20181120-what-if-a-deadly-influenza-pandemic-broke-out-today

Petric M, Comanor L, et al. 2006. "Role of the Laboratory in Diagnosis of Influenza During Seasonal Epidemics and Potential Pandemics." *Journal of Infectious Diseases* 194:S98–S110.

Potter CW. 2001. "A History of Influenza." *Journal of Applied Microbiology* 91:572–579.

Putri WCWS, Muscatello DJ, et al. 2018. "Economic Burden of Seasonal Influenza in the United States." *Vaccine* 36(27):3960–3966.

Rello J and Pop-Vicas A. 2009. "Clinical Review: Primary Influenza Viral Pneumonia." *Critical Care* 13(6):235.

Schenk AC and Shihadeh K. 2018. "Baloxavir Marboxil: A Novel Oral Antiviral Treatment for Uncomplicated Influenza." *Infectious Disease News* 31(12):7.

Schmid P, Rauber D, et al. 2017. "Barriers of Influenza Vaccination Intention and Behavior—A Systematic Review of Influenza Vaccine Hesitancy, 2005–2016." *PLoS ONE* 12(1). https://journals.plos.org/plosone/article?id=10.1371/journal.pone.0170550

Sellers SA, Hagan RS, et al. 2017. "The Hidden Burden of Influenza: A Review of the Extra-Pulmonary Complications of Influenza Infection." *Influenza and Other Respiratory Viruses* 11(5):372–393.

Smith TC. 2017. "Vaccine Rejection and Hesitancy: A Review and Call to Action." *Open Forum Infectious Diseases* 4(3). https://academic.oup.com/ofid/article/4/3/ofx146/3978712

Stanford Encyclopedia of Philosophy. 2012. *Empedocles.* https://plato.stanford.edu/entries/empedocles

Stulpin C. 2019. "'Common-Sense' Precautions Reduce Risk for Variant Flu at Fairs." *Infectious Disease News* 32(6):1, 12–14.

Stulpin C. 2020. "Worthwhile to Consider: Does the World Need a Pentavalent Flu Vaccine?" *Infectious Disease News* 33(1):1, 8.

Tatem AJ, Rogers DJ, et al. 2006. "Global Transport Networks and Infectious Disease Spread." *Advanced Parasitology* 6(62):293–343.

Taubenberger JK and Morens DM. 2006. "1918 Influenza: The Mother of All Pandemics." *Emerging Infectious Diseases* 12(1):15–22.

Thiel B. 2019. "Bad Flu Seasons Test US Hospitals." *Infectious Disease News* 32(2):1, 10–12.

Thorpe JR. 2016. "The Craziest Cures for the Flu in History." *Bustle.* https://www.bustle.com/articles/189943-the-craziest-cures-for-the-flu-in-history

U.S. Department of Health and Human Services, Centers for Disease Control and Prevention. 2018. *Influenza (Flu): Flu and You.* https://www.cdc.gov/flu/resource-center/freeresources/print/print-general.htm#FluandYou

Uyeki TM, Bernstein HH, et al. 2019. "Clinical Practice Guidelines by the Infectious Diseases Society of America: 2018 Update on Diagnosis, Treatment, Chemoprophylaxis, and Institutional Outbreak Management of Seasonal Influenza." *Clinical Infectious Diseases* 68(6):1–47.

Van Epps HL. 2006. "Influenza: Exposing the True Killer." *Journal of Experimental Medicine* 203:803.

Viboud C, Bjørnstad ON, et al. 2006. "Synchrony, Waves, and Spatial Hierarchies in the Spread of Influenza." *Science* 312(5772):447–451.

Walsh EE, Cox C, et al. 2002. "Clinical Features of Influenza A Virus Infection in Older Hospitalized Persons." *Journal of the American Geriatric Society* 50:1498–1503.

Waring JI. 1971. *A History of Medicine in South Carolina 1900–70.* Columbia, SC: South Carolina Medical Association.

Whitley RJ and Monto AS. 2006. "Prevention and Treatment of Influenza in High-Risk Groups: Children, Pregnant Women, Immunocompromised Hosts, and Nursing Home Residents." *Journal of Infectious Diseases* 194:S133–S138.

Whitley RJ and Monto AS. 2006. "Seasonal and Pandemic Influenza Preparedness: A Global Threat." *Journal of Infectious Diseases* 194:S65–S69.

Wong SS and Webby RJ. 2013. "Traditional and New Influenza Vaccines." *Clinical Microbiology Reviews* 26(3):476–492.

Yaqub O, Castle-Clarke S, et al. 2014. "Attitudes to Vaccination: A Critical Review." *Social Science & Medicine* 112:1–11.

Index

About the Author

R. K. Devlin is a practicing infectious diseases physician who lives near Lake Michigan in the Midwest. She received her medical degree from the University of Colorado, completed her residency in a combined Internal Medicine and Pediatrics program in Michigan, and finished her subspecialty training at Dartmouth. She is the author of several scientific papers and a previous book, *Influenza*. With an interest in reading and writing beyond the world of medicine, Dr. Devlin has also owned an independent bookstore, founded a literary nonprofit, and published numerous book reviews in online and print publications.